FIFTY SHADES

PHENOMENON

EXPLORING A SEXUAL REVOLUTION

FROM THE EDITORS OF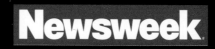

Media Lab Books
For inquiries, call 646-476-8860

Copyright 2015 Topix Media Lab

Published by Topix Media Lab
14 Wall Street, Suite 4B
New York, NY 10005

ISBN 10: 1-942556-00-4
ISBN-13: 978-1-942556-00-8

UNIVERSAL PICTURES AND FOCUS FEATURES

FIFTY SHADES OF WOMEN

From web-based sensation to global addiction, *Fifty Shades* is much more than a story: It's a movement.

It's shifted the sexual paradigm and has reshaped the way women everywhere approach and discuss their sexuality. Now, *Newsweek* explores the phenomenon that has fascinated and delighted women all over the world. With testimonials from people living the *Fifty* lifestyle, tips and tricks for heating things up in the bedroom and an exploration of the sexual revolution still underway, it's a comprehensive look at everything *Fifty*. Delving into every angle of this catalyst for a national conversation about lust, love, erotic fiction and the sacrifices that occur in any relationship, it's the definitive guide to America's hottest guilty pleasure. There's no doubt *Fifty Shades* has become a dominant force in our culture.

We're more than happy to submit to it.

Tie Breaker
In 2012, Brooks Brothers reported sales of neckties had increased 23 percent, no doubt a result of *Fifty*'s influence in bedrooms across the nation.

THE
FIFTY
PHENOMENON

EVOLUTION OF SEXY

How the "perfect man" has changed through the decades, from Clark Gable to James Dean and, now, to Christian Grey.

1920s
Rudolph Valentino
As Hollywood's first sex symbol, the Italian stud was so popular among women that the Sheik condom was named after his role in 1921's *The Sheik*.

1930s
Clark Gable
Best known for not giving a damn in 1939's *Gone With the Wind*, this suave, brooding man has been stealing women's hearts ever since. Scarlett can relate.

1940s
Cary Grant
Women wanted him and men wanted to be him (to which he replied, "So do I"), a reputation he upheld as cinema's debonair leading man.

1950s
James Dean
The phrase "teen heartthrob" was born with James Dean, courtesy of the actor's good looks, soulful eyes and unwavering ability to just play it cool.

1960s
Mick Jagger
The lead singer of The Rolling Stones and most popular frontman in the history of rock & roll will forever be known as a rule-breaking lady killer.

1970s
Burt Reynolds
The actor rose to sex-symbol fame after posing nearly nude for *Cosmopolitan* magazine and kept that momen-

1980s
Patrick Swayze
The beloved star of *Roadhouse* and *Dirty Dancing* knew all the right moves to dance his way into the hearts

1990s
Brad Pitt
His breakout role in *Legends of the Fall* secured his place in Hollywood, but Pitt's rugged, bad-boy

2000s
David Beckham
Whether stripping down to his skivvies to model for H&M or bending soccer balls to his will,

2015
Jamie Dornan
A new breed of sexy is born thanks to E L James's Christian Grey. The Irishman will become

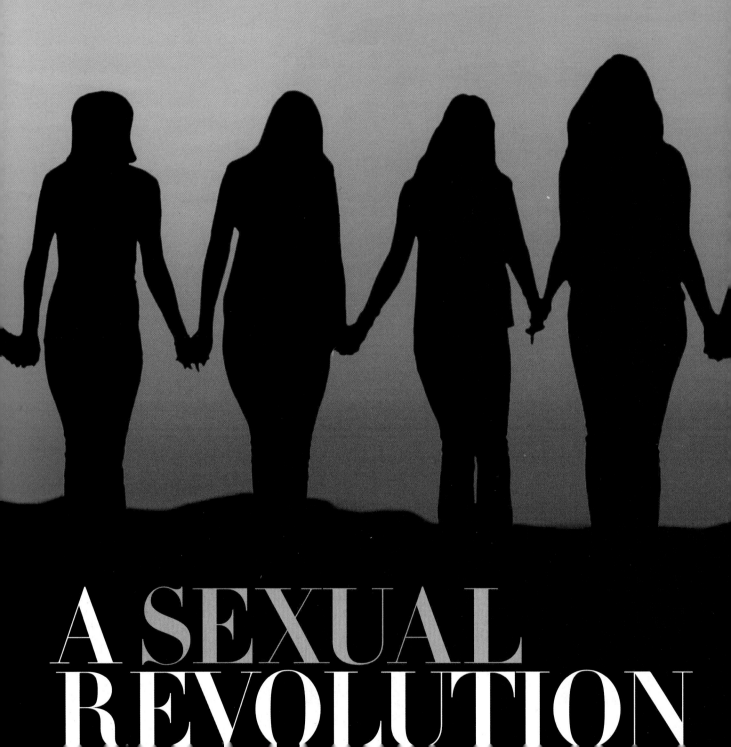

A SEXUAL REVOLUTION

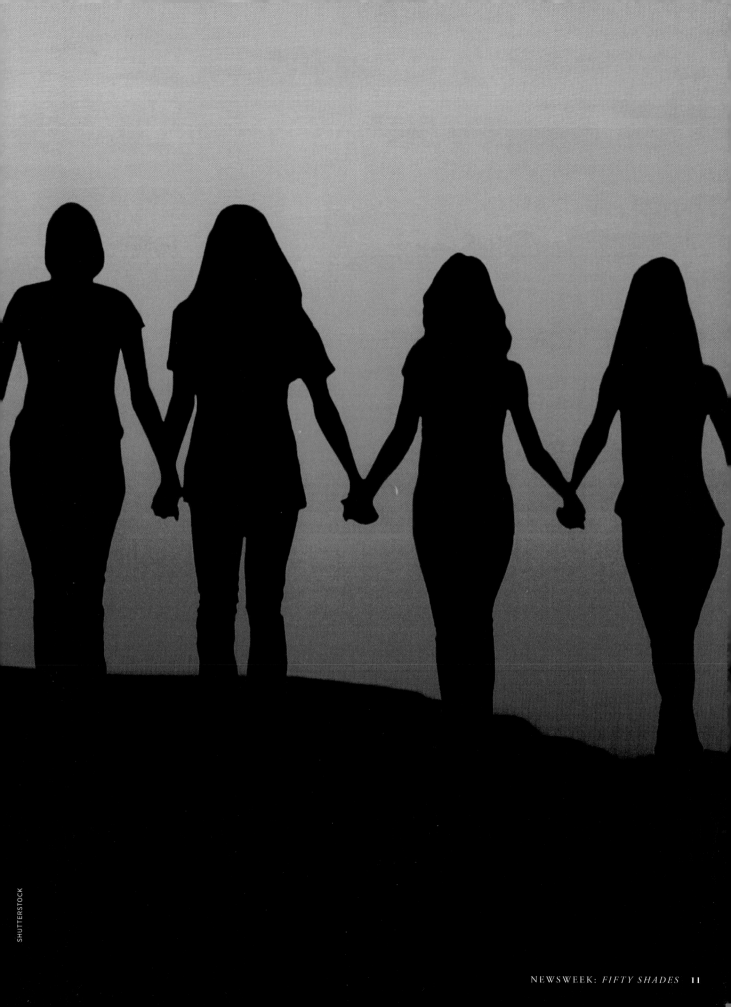

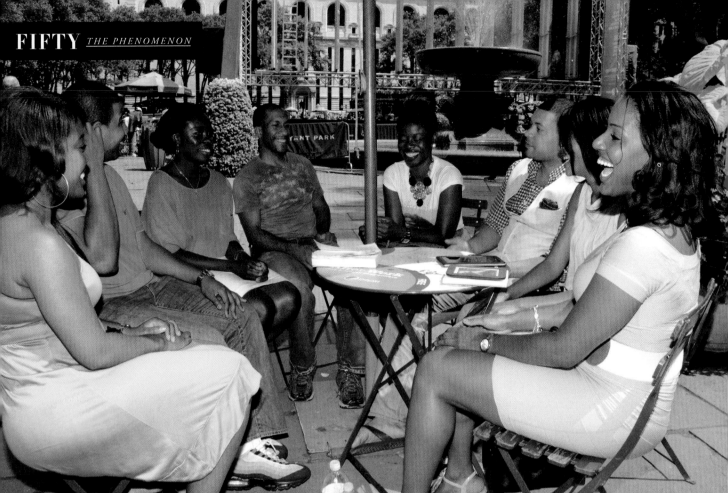

Fifty Fandom

Clockwise from top: Brunch and Books NYC meets every six weeks to enjoy a friendly meal and discuss a selected novel, one of which was *Fifty Shades of Grey*; a book signing in New York in 2012 included a knot tying contest; E L James's *Fifty Shades*-inspired wine collection.

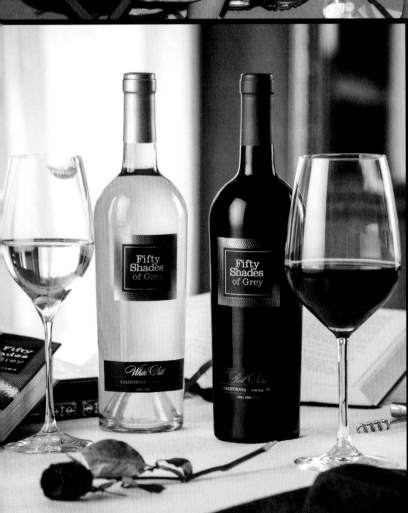

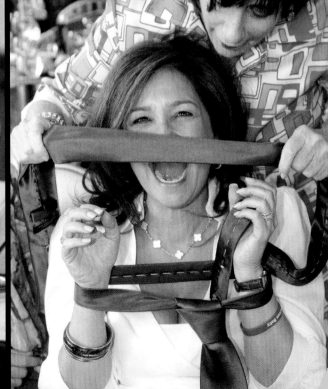

Fifty Shades of Grey became a cultural phenomenon not because it was heavily advertised or because it was required reading at every school in America. It became popular the old-fashioned way: People read it, liked it and told their friends, who in turn told their friends, who told their moms, who told their hairstylists and so on. Erotica has always been recommended over the back fence, woman to woman. But in the age of social media, sharing your opinion about a book you couldn't put down no longer means telling your five closest friends; it means tweeting about it to your 500 followers.

The series, which found its way into mainstream publishing from the online world of *Twilight* fan fiction, has sold more than 100 million copies since its release in May 2011, surpassing the sales of *Harry Potter*. The film's Facebook page at time of publication had 6.7 million likes, up 5 million from just a year prior. It also has Twitter and Instagram accounts with a combined 400,000 followers, plus a presence on Pinterest and YouTube. An official app, the Grey Enterprises Internship Program, launched in January 2014, offering activities and incentives for members (open to all) who are rewarded with exclusive content and sneak peeks of the film. There's *Fifty Shades* nail polish, makeup, wine and, as if on cue, lingerie and sex toys. Needless to say, word has gotten around, and the humble work of Snowqueen's Icedragon (E L James's original nom de plume) has become a full blown phenomenon. Not bad for a smutty novel criticized for its purple prose, unbelievable characters and cheesy wish-fulfillment.

"I've seen better storytelling in an evening news segment about a raccoon who got a peanut butter jar stuck on his head in a Wendy's parking lot," wrote Julieanne Smolinski in a 2012 *Vulture* review. She's hardly alone in her opinion. But whether people are bashing it or gushing over it, *The New York Times*, *TIME* magazine, the *Today* show, small-town newspapers and (probably) even your grandmother's book club all rode the hype, openly discussing *Fifty Shades of Grey* and running stories about why suburban housewives were suddenly reading erotica—or at least openly admitting to it. One *New York Times* columnist asked his Twitter followers to suggest the male equivalent of a woman reading *Fifty*

> *"In today's climate, more than giving women something to talk about, some people see Fifty Shades as giving women permission to talk, period."*

Shades on the subway. Answers varied, from *Playboy* and the *Sports Illustrated Swimsuit Issue* to anything by Dan Brown.

Despite dismissals of the book as a passing fad and quippy comments about "mommy porn"—a term that E L James has said she finds "disparaging"—the author's inner goddess is doing backflips. And so is her inner accountant: James's net worth is currently estimated at $80 million.

But more than the economic stimulus the book created for James and booksellers, it also stimulated the collective sex drive of women around the world. A 2013 study by luxury sex toy brand LELO found that sales of wearable toys and massagers increased by 82 percent. LELO surveyed 25,000 people and found that though the trend of BDSM seemed to be plateauing in 2014 as more women return

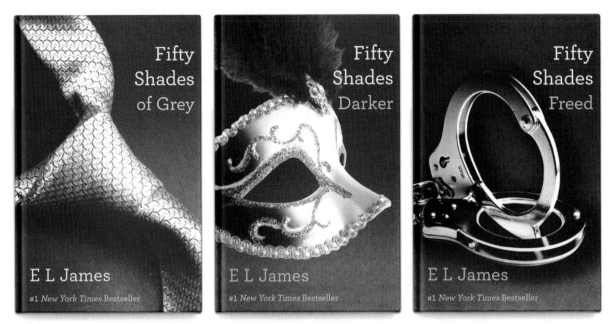

Selling Sensation *Fifty Shades of Grey* flew off the shelves following its May 2011 release, increasing Barnes & Noble's revenue by 2 percent. Like any blockbuster, it has sequels.

to "vanilla" sex, their confident and adventurous sides have skyrocketed, and with anticipation of the film growing, those trends could easily shift again come February 14, 2015.

The book has also sparked a global dialogue between wives and husbands, therapists and patients, even mothers and daughters. It's opened the figurative doors for conversation among women about what goes on behind their literal ones. Standard book-of-the-month clubs have been revived with the welcome integration of wine, cheese and recaps of steamy scenes from novels the members have all read together.

It's also reinvigorated the cultural debate over who defines women's sexuality. Here, *Fifty Shades'* popularity might be a function of good timing. In today's climate, more than giving women something to talk about, some people see *Fifty Shades* as giving women permission to talk, period.

"We live in a society that essentially caters to men's desires, as much as we try to make things egalitarian," says Avital Norman Nathman, a renowned feminist writer and blogger for *The Mamafesto*. "It's not really wholly surprising when people are up in arms the moment a woman expresses some sort of desire."

But when you get down to the nuts and bolts of what truly makes this book so popular,

people still find themselves stumped. Why *Fifty Shades of Grey*? Men are certainly confused. In a world that's always had trouble figuring out exactly what women want from guys, Christian's penchant for stalking and spanking goes against the values of equality heralded by modern society.

Women are equally stumped. Female fans cite the engrossing love story, Christian and Ana's fantasy life and the simple need to know what happens next. But for every blogger or expert proclaiming *Fifty Shades* an emancipating tool for women, there's another decrying it as dangerous trash.

A new study published in an August 2014 edition of the *Journal of Women's Health* found *Fifty Shades of Grey* readers are more likely to have verbally abusive partners and exhibit signs of eating disorders than those who haven't read the books. Lead researcher of the study, Dr. Amy Bonomi, argues that the books "perpetuate dangerous abuse standards" and romanticize dangerous behavior.

The author herself doesn't seem too worked up over all the fuss: "I just wrote it as my midlife crisis, really," James told a New Zealand television station. But however modest her intentions, there's no denying that E L James has started a conversation that's blossomed into a full-blown revolution. And it doesn't seem to be dying down anytime soon.

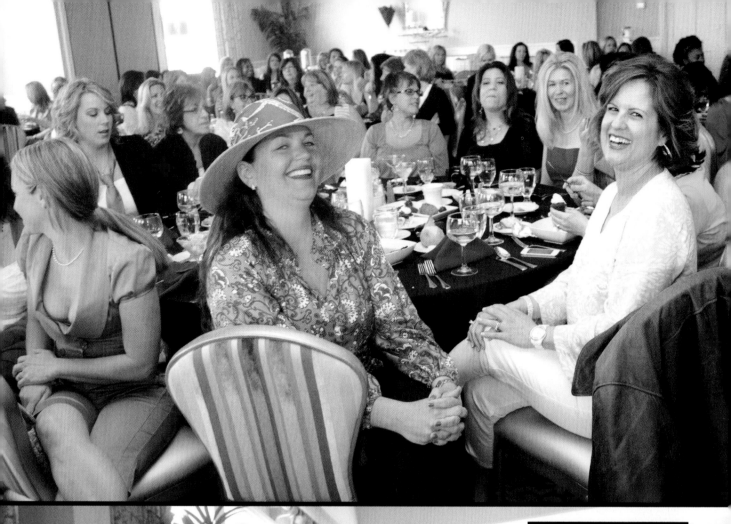

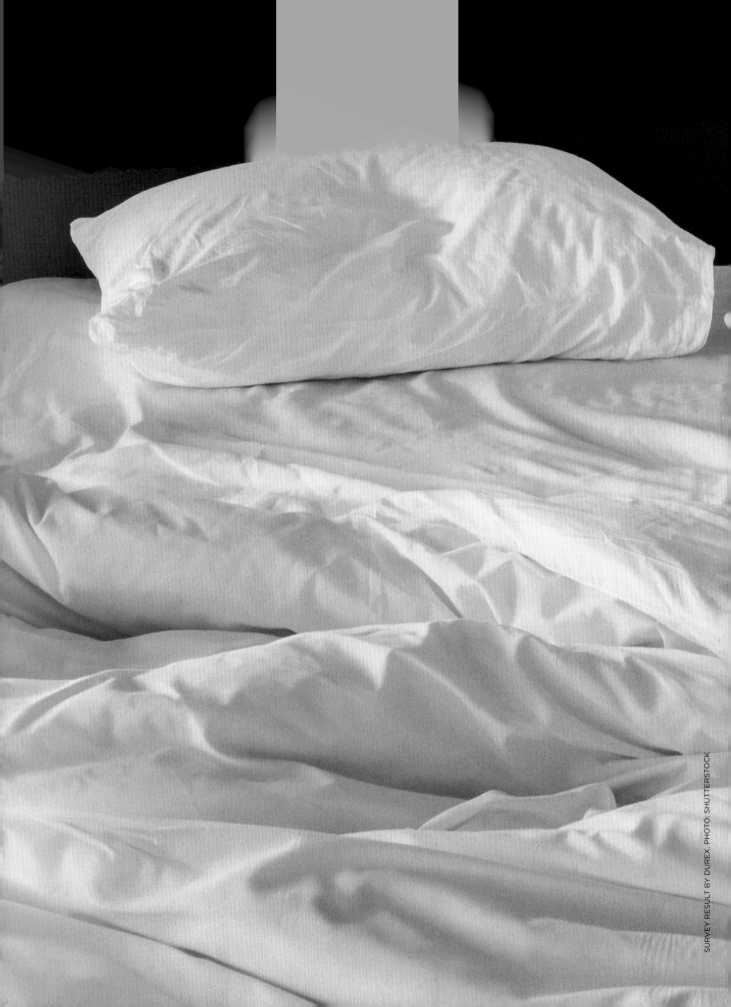

46% of Americans believe it's more likely they'll see BigFoot than "finish" at the same time as their partner.

THE FIFTY CREATOR

A look at the modest life of erotica's surprising savior.

E rika Leonard is just like you. She's flirty, funny and a little camera shy. In fact, the biggest difference between Leonard and you is that, using the pseudonym E L James, she wrote a book that changed the way women globally perceive (and approach) sexuality.

The transition from late-40s working mom to S&M guru for the sexually frustrated can be jarring, even if the volumes happen to be made up of one's own most vivid sexual fantasies. But how exactly did mild-mannered BBC television producer Erika Leonard become E L James, master of the erotica universe?

Born in London to a Chilean mother and a Scottish father, Leonard studied history at the University of Kent before entering the television business as a manager's assistant at the National Film and Television School in London. She met her husband (and soon-to-be erotica test dummy) while employed at the school. The couple have been married for nearly 30 years and have two sons. Mr. Leonard, who described himself in *The Guardian* as "the least romantic [person] who ever lived," has appeared on British television and said that the couple's sex life is not the basis for Ana and Christian's. But, James has also let slip that her husband was tired out by the primary research for the novels.

Over the course of an extensive career in TV production, Leonard developed quite the CV, working on projects as diverse as *There's Only One Madonna*, which traced the pop superstar's career from its beginnings to her 2001 Drowned World Tour, and *Bodies*, an hour-long BBC medical drama.

After reading Stephenie Meyer's *Twilight* series, Leonard was moved to write her own take on the story. She became "Snowqueen's Icedragon," the moniker she used to publish an early version of *Fifty Shades of Grey*, titled "Master of the Universe," in an online fan fiction forum.

Before *Fifty Shades* made the transition to print, Leonard needed a pen name rather than a screen name and arrived at "E L James" without much difficulty. "To be honest, I didn't give it a huge amount of thought," she told *The Boston Globe* in 2012. "In three minutes I thought of E L James." James is a family name, E is her first initial and L is her middle initial, though Leonard won't disclose what it stands for.

As E L James, Erika Leonard has given the book publishing industry a much needed boost. Her original book deal was worth six figures, to say

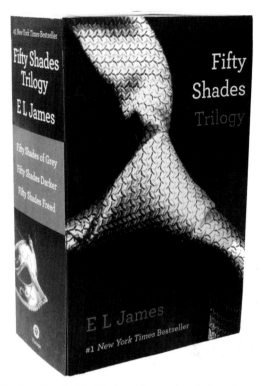

The Fifty Effect *Fifty Shades of Grey* took only 11 weeks to sell 1 million copies after hitting shelves, breaking the record of 36 weeks previously set by Dan Brown's *The Da Vinci Code*.

nothing of the fact her earnings between June 2012 and June 2013 rang in at $95 million. By all accounts, the money has yet to change Leonard's day-to-day life, however, as the author has been known to shop at IKEA and wrestled with the cost of a pair of £110 Ugg boots.

Despite her modest lifestyle, writing one of the most popular books in history has garnered her a feature film, set to release on Valentine's Day. Though the author was hesitant to dive into the world of film adaptation, she told *Entertainment Weekly* last year, "I thought, 'I'm middle-aged; when in the hell am I going to get another chance to make a movie in Hollywood?' " Leonard embraced the film adaptation right away, complete with script approval, casting credit and a constant presence on set in Vancouver.

But as fans impatiently wait for the big screen reveal, they can do so with this little bit of hope: Leonard has written another book. When or if that book will make it to print is still undetermined, though she has admitted that it's nothing like *Fifty Shades of Grey*.

What is known for certain, however, is that the characters she created in her first novel have lived on longer than she could ever have imagined. And women all over the world love her for it.

WELCOME TO FIFTY SHADES FUNLAND

Move over, Potter. There's a new theme park in the works guaranteed to be a hit with you and your mate! When everyday life has you feeling tied down, escape to this playground of pleasure (and pain).

ILLUSTRATION BY **KYLE HILTON**

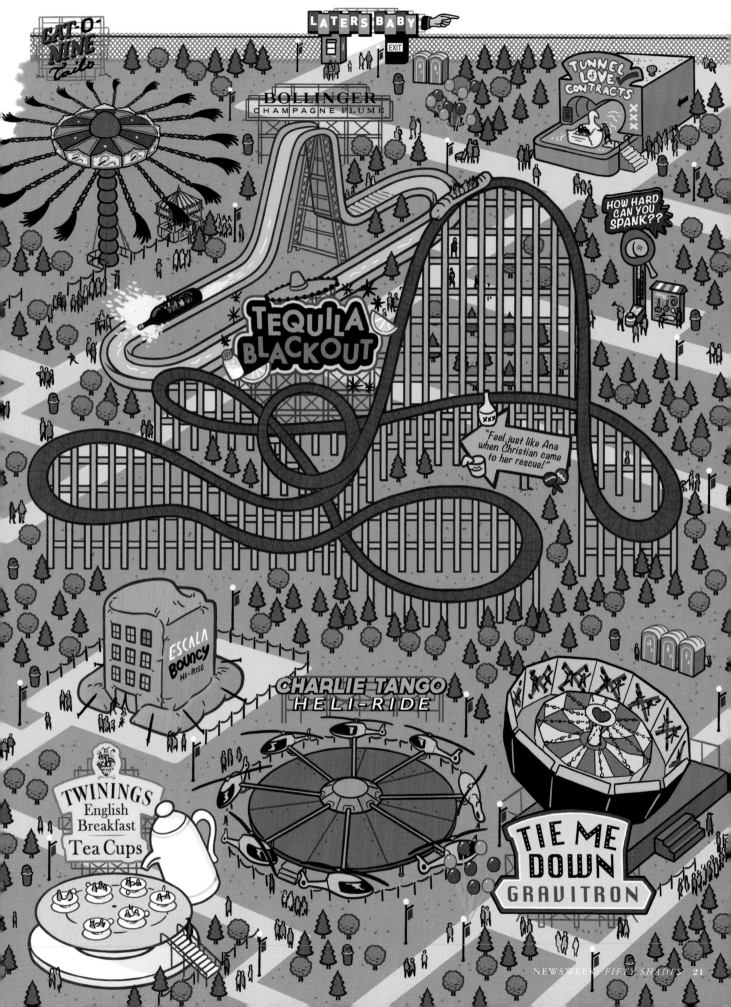

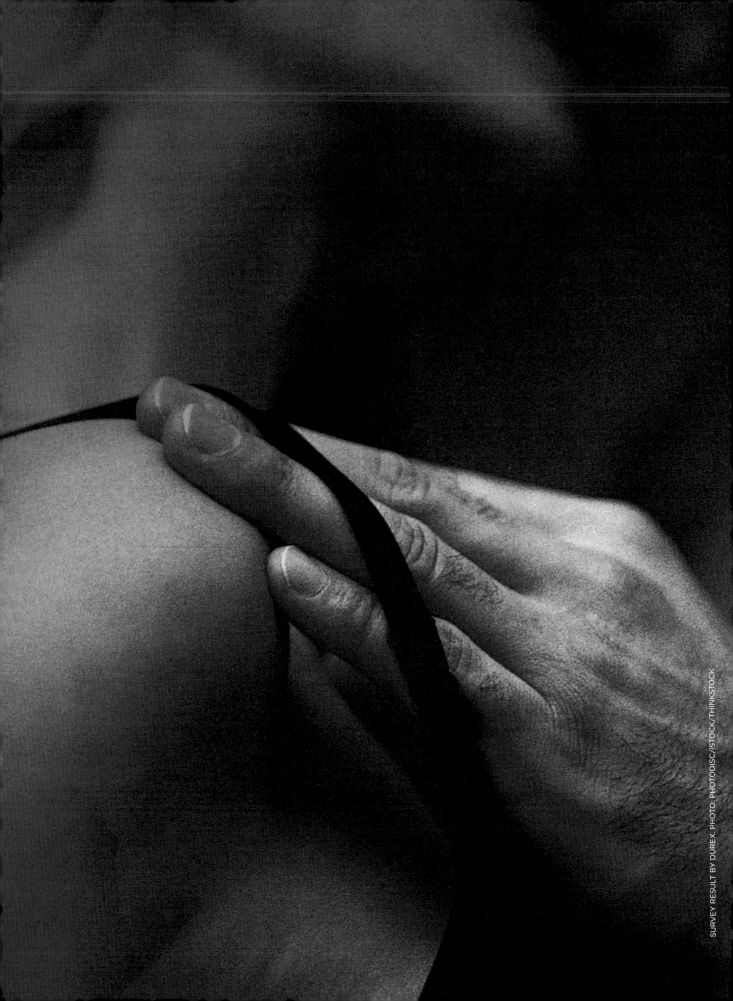

87% of women said the hottest sex they've had was with someone they trusted.

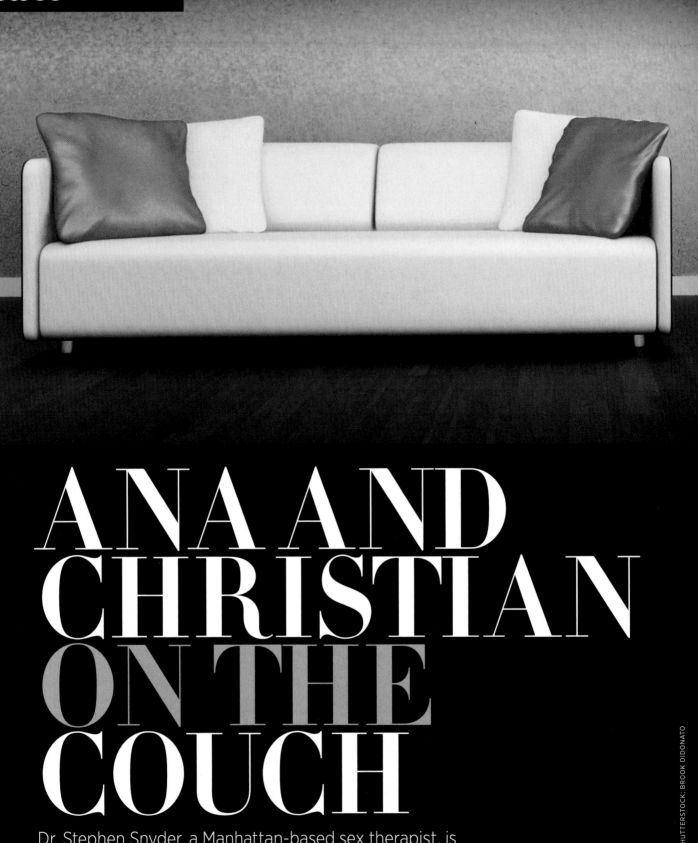

ANA AND CHRISTIAN ON THE COUCH

Dr. Stephen Snyder, a Manhattan-based sex therapist, is a bigger fan of *Fifty Shades of Grey* than you are, though his reasons are clinical in nature.

What do you like about *Fifty Shades of Grey*?
I like that it's sexual fantasy, and it works. Since it's popular, everyone has permission to read it. Many sex therapists have found if you give *Fifty Shades* to one or both members of a couple, sometimes it sparks something.

In what ways is Ana and Christian's relationship healthy?
Well, it's fiction, so one can't read too much into it. But I like that Ana and Christian each stay completely true to what they need—even when their needs are in collision. Serious conflict always occurs in a relationship, sooner or later. And when it does, you have three choices. You can break up. You can just go on as if the problem doesn't exist. Or you can face it while holding true to your needs—usually this means suffering together until, through your own willingness to go beyond yourselves, you eventually find your way as a couple. That's what Christian and Ana do in the book. And *Fifty Shades* captures something of the agony and the ecstasy of the process.

In what ways is it unhealthy?
It's important to keep in mind that sexual domination is different from emotional domination. Being sexually dominated, or fantasizing about it, can be a great turn-on. But being emotionally dominated is ordinarily just abusive. Ana seems to understand the difference. She has no interest in being emotionally dominated, and she makes sure Christian knows it. But she's an idealized fictional character. She's well-educated, psychologically very strong and economically independent. Many real women aren't so lucky. For most, it would be a serious mistake to get involved with such an emotionally dominating man. Most men like that won't change—not even after three volumes of great sex.

By bringing "non-vanilla" sexual themes into the mainstream, do you think *Fifty Shades* has made things like bondage passé?
It might have made bondage seem more ordinary. Eros needs to be situated somewhere

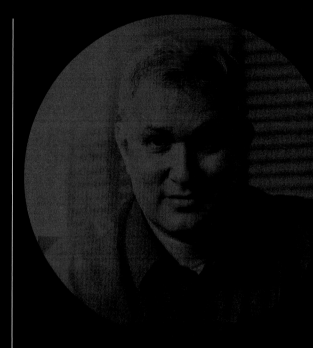

Dr. Snyder is a sex and relationship specialist with 25 years of experience and is an Associate Clinical Professor of Psychiatry at the Mount Sinai School of Medicine.

between the safe and the transgressive. Early on in a relationship, simply being naked together can feel like a transgression—a breaking down of the usual social barriers. Later on, many couples complain about the lack of any transgressive thrill. I encourage couples to keep taking risks with each other. Usually this involves emotional risks—telling each other things you would ordinarily keep private. But sexual risks are important too.

Short of becoming a young, self-made millionaire, how can a guy become more like Christian?
Christian is a master glider pilot, sailor, sexual dominant and above all a master capitalist. That sense of mastery is often very, very appealing to women. But every man can be a master at something. It doesn't have to be anything so glamorous. When a man takes quiet pride in the places where he truly is a master, that can have real erotic value. Women, let yourselves enjoy the realms where your partner has mastery. Hopefully it's something other than video games.

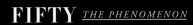

CAN YOU ACTUALLY CHANGE A MAN?

Ana managed to change Christian without driving him away. Can other women do the same? Dr. Christina Villarreal has answers.

For starters, can a guy even be changed?
Yes. The bottom line is there has to be incentive. He's got to be getting something out of it, too.

Rather than waking him at 2 a.m. to yell about the toilet seat being up, when should you tell him you're mad? 4 a.m.?
Only if your goal is to make him angry. Also, you shouldn't raise the topic of change while you two are arguing or when he's at work. That never goes over well. Wait until you have some face-to-face time with him.

What if he doesn't see that something's wrong? What do we do?
Don't let his behavior get under your skin. Feel confident that you're bringing something that he wants to the table. Don't sit down and wallow in sadness because you think your relationship is going down the drain. Go out and get your needs met elsewhere. We're always going to have something that men want, and if they want it, they're going to work for it. But you have to make them work for it.

Is it a good plan to trade sexual favors for a positive change in behavior?
Absolutely! Either doing what he wants or withholding are perfectly legitimate tactics in a relationship.

Can hooking up with someone else solve the problem?
I can't endorse cheating as an answer, but you should have a backup plan. Call it a Plan B. Tell the boyfriend who is totally slacking, "There are other options than you, and you're not the only man who is ever going to want me." A woman should feel empowered and not keep a guy around if he's acting like a [jerk].

When do we end it?
If he's spending a lot of time around other women, he's already telling you he's checked out of the relationship. It's on you to believe him and leave. If he's constantly criticizing what you're eating or how you look, that's 100 percent grounds for a breakup. Move on! There will be another guy who likes how you look.

"We're always going to have something that men want, and if they want it, they're going to work for it."

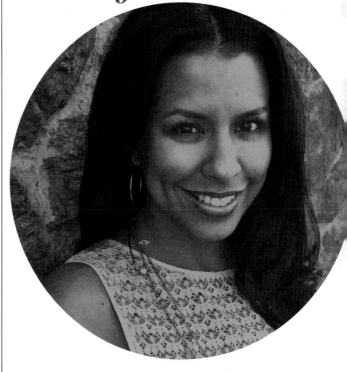

Dr. Villarreal is a clinical psychologist based in San Francisco, California, focused on helping people with mental health issues, relationship difficulties and sexual exploration problems.

96% OF MEN AGREE SATISFYING THEIR PARTNERS **COMES BEFORE BEING SATISFIED THEMSELVES**

"I remember the moment *I knew you were the one."* —The phrase that gets women turned on the quickest.

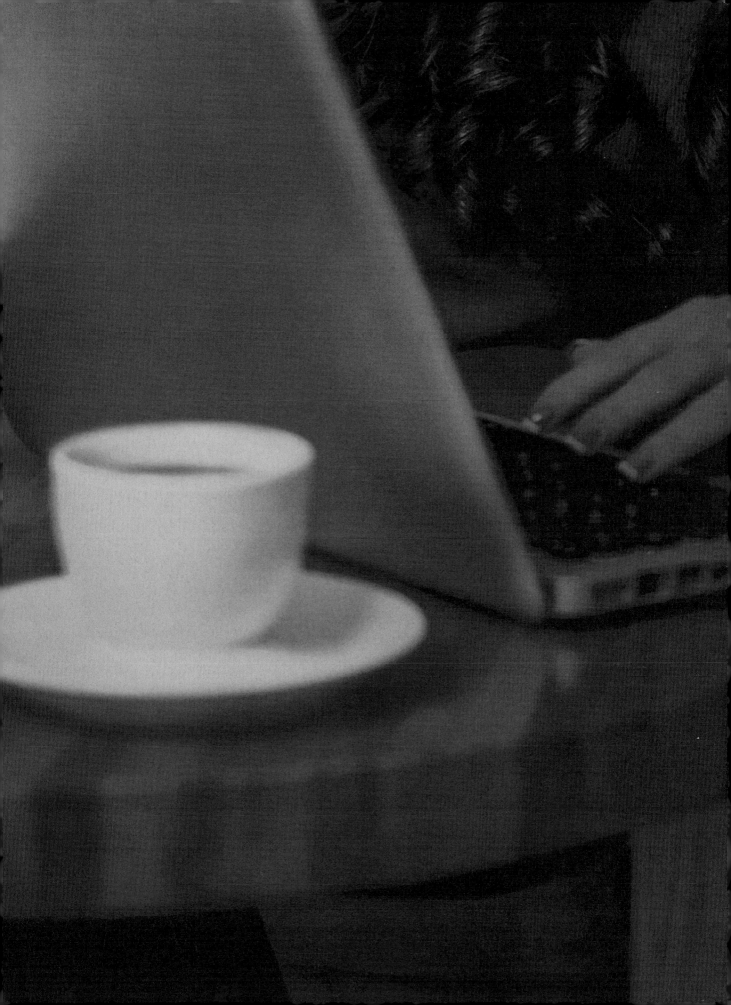

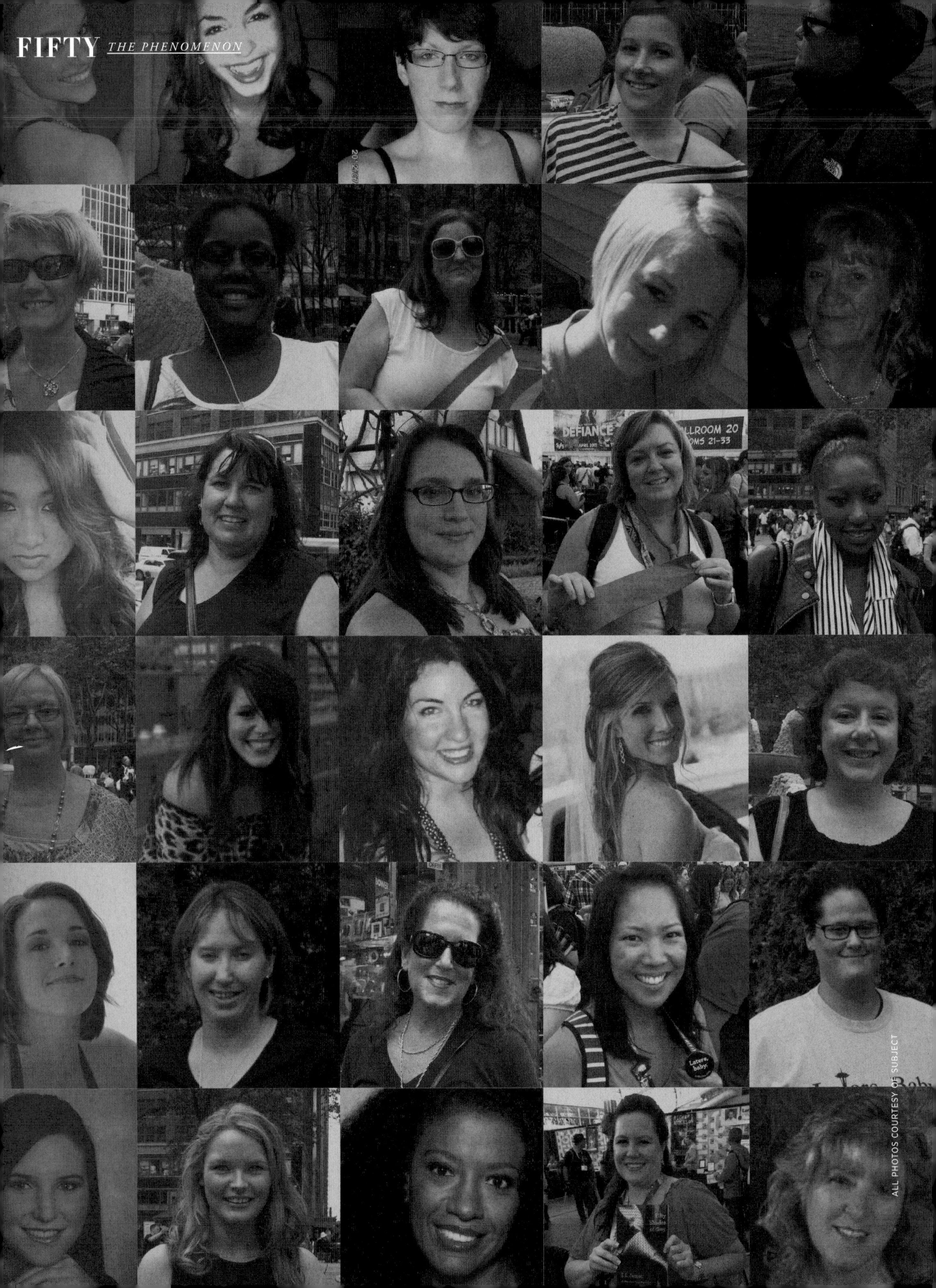

ALL PHOTOS COURTESY OF SUBJECT

FIFTY
SHADES
OF WOMEN

Real stories from fans just like you.

TARA, 28
New York, NY

My fiancé and I had a mishap with some candle play. We were like "Ooo fun! Sexy candles!" Maybe we poured it on too fast, but we had it lit, and we poured it on my stomach and I was like, "F***!" You put it on your stomach, and it's hot, and you can't pull it off, because it's STILL HOT, so I got burned. I don't know if it was a poorly designed candle, or if we just didn't do it right. Might have been a bit of both. It didn't kill the mood. I just told him not to touch my stomach.

HEIDI, 51
STEPHENS POINT, WI
WAS ANA A LITTLE ANNOYING? SURE. DID I CARE? NOT A DAMN BIT.

MARLIE, 27
Los Angeles, CA

I was flying from Florida back to L.A. and had a few friends that were kind of ranting about it, so I figured that since everyone was talking about it, I'd pick one up. It's very imaginative...like, "Wow, can you really do that?" I will say it's made reading a lot more fun.

SUE, 33
New Jersey

BDSM has always been appealing to me, but I've found it difficult to find a man that is open-minded enough to try it. It seems this book is making it easier to find that. I can't tell you the amount of male friends that have been commenting, "My wife is reading *Fifty Shades*...I haven't had this much sex in years." My female friends have asked me for advice on

CATHERINE, 29
NEW YORK, NY

The books aren't exactly genius, so some friends of mine were surprised I was reading them. The funniest reaction was from a woman I babysit for. Her daughter had gone to bed so it wasn't like I was talking to her child about the book or anything. But I didn't get a sense of judgment from her about it. It was more like she was shocked I wasn't making any sort of effort to protect my privacy. She said, "You're not even trying to hide it?" I thought that was funny. It was one of the first conversations I've had where I was aware that my reading *Fifty Shades* sends a message that I'm a sexual human being. But it's like, "Of course I am! Why wouldn't I be?" I haven't been asked to do anything in BDSM, but I wouldn't necessarily turn it down outright, and I think that does have to do with reading the book. I didn't know I was open to being tied up and ordered around, for example. I'm open to sexual activity I wasn't necessarily open to before, so maybe in that way the books are genius.

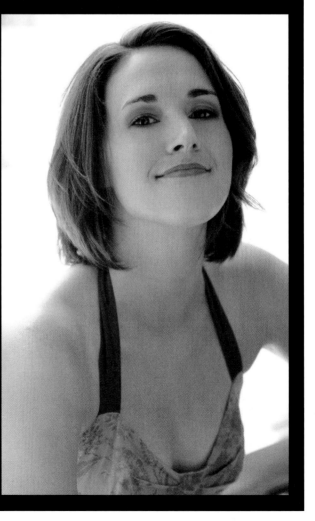

incorporating aspects of BDSM into their sex lives. They knew I was into unconventional things, but none knew the extent.

DEB, 30
Stamford, CT

Apparently, there's a *Fifty Shades* "baby boom" underway from all the women who had a spark in their sex lives, so it's pretty crazy how much this book has affected the world! Cake decorating is my side job, and I always try to attend fun celebrity events with cakes that replicate the product being promoted. A friend and I decided to go to the book signing with a *Fifty Shades* book cake and themed cupcakes to give to E L James when we had our

CHRISTIAN DOESN'T LIVE IN SEATTLE. IF HE DID, I WOULD HAVE FOUND HIM AND LOCKED HIM IN MY BASEMENT BY NOW.
JULIA, 38 // SEATTLE, WA

AFTER GAINING WEIGHT AND FEELING UNCOMFORTABLE ABOUT MYSELF, I STOPPED WANTING TO HAVE SEX WITH MY HUSBAND. I THEN STARTED READING THE BOOKS AND, AS THEY SAY, IT GOT MY JUICES FLOWING. MY HUSBAND HAS BEEN A LOT HAPPIER.
NAOMI, 37 // UNITED KINGDOM

books signed. She was the sweetest!

BETSY, 43
New York, NY

It's hard to feel sexy when you're packing lunch and doing laundry. Being able to conjure up how scenes from the book affected me made our marriage more passionate. My husband calls *Fifty Shades of Grey* the best book he's never read.

BINCY, 20
Troy, MI

It was all over my Facebook feed, so that got me interested. I literally read it within a week. But it was really shocking. I didn't even know BDSM existed! I didn't know anything about a dominant or a submissive or that people were actually into stuff like that.

MARUSKA, 41
UNITED KINGDOM

EVERYBODY WATCHES PORN, EVERYBODY DOES CRAZY, KINKY THINGS AND, YOU KNOW, IT'S CRAZY FOR PEOPLE TO SAY BAD THINGS ABOUT IT. IF YOU HAVEN'T TRIED IT, DON'T MOCK IT.

JOAN, 68
Sebastopol, CA

I would say that this book is not a huge phenomenon in my age group; however, there are plenty reading it. If you read the Amazon reviews, which are delightful to read, they're really funny.

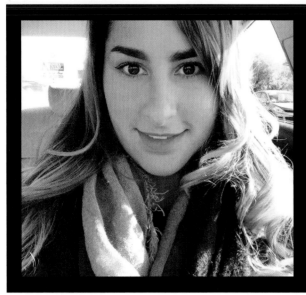

LAURA, 25
N. PROVIDENCE, RI

I never knew some of the things Christian used and did even *existed*. I only started reading *Fifty Shades* because I needed to understand what all the hype was about. I hopped right on the bandwagon. I couldn't put it down! I took it everywhere with me. It was very compelling and informative. My boss had to have a "talk" with me for reading it at work. He was not intrigued at all. If only he knew!

One man said, "I'm in my 70s. I take Viagra just to read it." We are not so easily shocked because we've been around the block and the other block. Lots of blocks, really. And we may have experienced different things in our own sexuality or just have had the opportunity to meet more people and talk to them. We're not so easily shocked, and we definitely like to be titillated. People in my age group are also reading, if I may say, better erotica. There's a lot of better erotica than *Fifty Shades*, but the phenomenon is pretty amazing.

LYDIA, 37
Worcester, MA

I'm a single mom and I work, I go to school, I'm a very busy person. But I actually had to call an old "friend with benefits"

after I read the book because I was just like...well...you know.

JENNY, 35
Vancouver, British Columbia, Canada

I'd be lying if I said it hasn't changed my sex life. There's a reason romance novels, especially erotica, have been popular for so long even if it hasn't been considered mainstream. My husband and I have been together for more than 17 years. It is important to keep things interesting.

LUCY, 42
Boise, ID

I enjoyed reading *Fifty Shades*, but I think I've enjoyed the side effects of reading it more. The sex with my husband has been better. I'm not saying it was bad before, I'm just saying it's been better. He hasn't read the books, he just knows I have. I can't tell if it's because I'm more in the mood, or if my husband feels like he's competing with a fictional character so he upped his game. Either way, let it be known: I'm not complaining.

ELIZABETH, 26
MONTEREY, CA
I WAS SO ENTHRALLED BY IT THAT I ENDED UP READING IT ON MY NOOK WHILE MY BOYFRIEND'S PARENTS WERE IN TOWN. IN FRONT OF THEM. THEY HAD NO IDEA.

WHEN I FOUND OUT MY MOM HAD READ IT, I WAS A LITTLE SURPRISED. THEN I HEARD MY DAD WAS THE ONE WHO RECOMMENDED IT.
TERI, 29 // ROANOKE, VA

ALL MY FRIENDS HAVE READ IT, BUT I THINK I'M THE ONLY ONE WHO'S READ IT 12 TIMES.
SHEREE, 22 // KANSAS CITY, MO

SAMANTHA, 31
AUSTIN, TX
MY SEX LIFE POST-*FIFTY SHADES* HASN'T CHANGED MUCH, BUT MY DATING LIFE HAS. I'VE ALREADY BEEN OUT WITH THREE HELICOPTER PILOTS!

ERIKA, 22
Gulfport, MS

I used to think that being a mom meant I couldn't do things like that in the bedroom, that parents shouldn't do that kind of thing. But now I feel the bedroom is a place for you and your spouse to have fun, explore each other and escape from everyday life. *Fifty Shades* gave me the courage to explore my boundaries and also changed the way I look at every Audi I see on the street!

LAUREN, 28
Alpharetta, GA
I went on a blind date with a guy who noticed the book in my bag. He was like, "I can be that guy." He seemed a little mysterious, and he was kind of cute, so I agreed to go back to his place. He had three roommates and a twin bed. I didn't stick around long enough to find out if he could cook an omelette.

KATIE, 19
Orlando, FL
At first, I was a little shocked. But one thing I got out of the book is knowing that you have to have limits, but even with those limits, when the right person comes along, it's OK to let them push your limits a little.

ELISE, 26
MESA, AZ
I'LL SAY THIS: THE RIDING CROP THING TURNED ME ON. AND THEN I TRIED IT AND QUICKLY REALIZED THAT I'M A BIG BABY AND DON'T LIKE BEING HIT WITH ANYTHING. IT'S HARD TO BE SEXY WHEN YOU'RE CRYING. THAT GUY HASN'T CALLED ME SINCE.

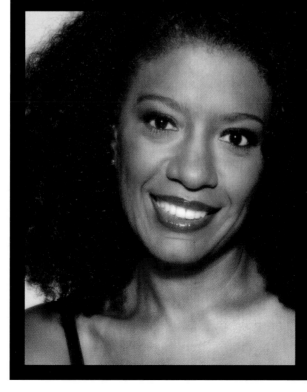

HELEN, 50
NEW YORK, NY
I've bought the book for other people! For the first two weeks after finishing the last book, it was so much a part of my routine, and that routine was gone. I missed the routine, and I missed knowing what was going on in their lives. I was on my way to work when I saw an Audi, I think it was an R8—you don't see a lot of them on the road here. I thought, "Oh my God. I wonder if that's some billionaire's girlfriend!"

I'M ON MY THIRD COPY. I LEFT ONE ON A PLANE AND DROPPED THE OTHER IN THE TUB. I WAS DISTRACTED BOTH TIMES, FOR DIFFERENT REASONS.
ALICE, 28 // CHICAGO, IL

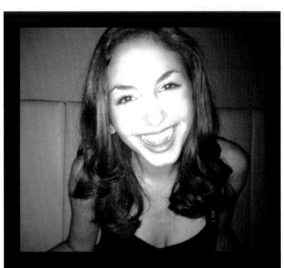

CHRISTIAN'S NO PUSH-OVER. "WHATEVER MAKES YOU HAPPY—" NO. HE'S A MAN, AND I THINK THAT WOMEN FIND THAT VERY ATTRACTIVE: A MAN WHO TAKES WHAT HE WANTS. THERE'S SOMETHING VERY PRIMAL AND SEXY ABOUT THAT.
ALI, 19 // NEW YORK, NY

HELENA, 44
PORTLAND, ME
I'D BE LYING IF I SAID IT DIDN'T TURN ME ON. I'D ALSO BE LYING IF I TOLD YOU MY HUSBAND AND I HAVEN'T WRITTEN UP OUR OWN LITTLE SEX CONTRACT!

ANGEL, 37
Trenton, NJ

There was one night where my husband and I went through, chapter by chapter, and highlighted the passages that we each enjoyed, like a wish list. I highlighted a lot of the sexy parts. He highlighted the scene where they go gliding. So I highlighted the part where Christian says he makes $100,000 an hour. He said to find out how much riding crops cost.

DEBORAH, 19
Newark, NJ

I posted a status on Facebook after I'd gone halfway through the book that said, "This is so unreal. I can't believe what I'm reading right now." And within 30 seconds of posting, I got poked by this big womanizer from my school. He was older than me, and we never talked in high school, so I thought it was a mistake and I ignored it. Two minutes later, he starts messaging me, "That relationship, that's real, that happens in real life. It's a really ideal way to have a relationship," and all this stuff. We got into a conversation about what an ideal relationship is. He was saying, "Maybe you haven't found the right person to do that with. It's a lot more intimate, and the love is a lot stronger in those kinds of relationships." I said I wouldn't be opposed to trying it. Honestly, everybody that reads this book gets a little curious. He said we should keep talking as I read the book, and when I told him I'd

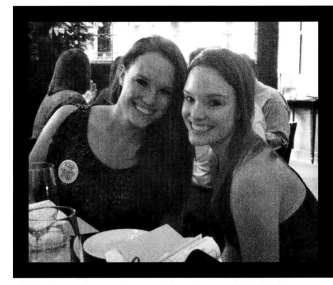

Ashley My mother was reading it, and I was like, "I don't want to have these images in my head!" But Alex and I talk about it a little just because we're very open with each other.

Alex Talking about it with my family wasn't that awkward. It's not like I was talking about my personal experience with any of this stuff. The only awkward part was when my mother found out my boyfriend was the one who bought it for me.

finished it, he started sending me very explicit pictures of himself. It was incredibly surprising and out of the blue. I don't really want any more to do with him now.

REXANA, 58
Elkhart, IN

I have friends who wouldn't touch it with a 10-foot pole, but I read it in less than 24 hours. I went right from one to the next and didn't quit until I read them all. I waited a couple

days, then said, "Maybe I should go back through and see what I missed and skipped when I was getting to the hot, steamy parts."

EFFIE, 41
Toronto, ON, Canada

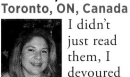 I didn't just read them, I devoured them. I'd stay up until 3 a.m. I could not put this novel down. I felt I could connect with Ana. My husband is not a reader. He's

into action, he's more of a doer. But I convinced him to read the end of *Fifty Shades Freed*, where it's Christian's point of view. I was curious to see if he would respond to that better as opposed to it being from Anastasia's point of view. And the funny thing was he was like, "OK, yeah, I read it. But I still would rather do it than read it." And of course my eyebrow cocked up all the way to my hairline and I thought, "This is going to be fun."

DEBI, 37
Oklahoma City, OK

 Christian's so attentive but also sort of the bad boy. Everybody likes the mysterious "don't really know what he's gonna do next" part. And obviously the billionaire part doesn't hurt either!

MELISSA, 33
AKRON, OH
THERE WEREN'T MANY SCENES THAT SHOCKED ME. EXCEPT MAYBE [SPOILER ALERT] WHEN ANA LEFT HIM IN THE END. I'D HAVE SIGNED THAT CONTRACT DAY ONE.

I HOPE WOMEN CAN TAKE IT AS AN OPPORTUNITY TO TAKE CONTROL OF WHAT THEY WANT, NO PUN INTENDED.
CAROLINE, 25 // NEW YORK, NY

LINDSAY, 29
Charleston, SC

I work in a pharmacy, and lately we've been seeing a lot of girls come in with UTIs and yeast infections. A lot more than usual. We finally got to the bottom of it...a lot of these girls were recreating the infamous ice cream scene in *Fifty Shades Darker*, which, though kind of sexy on paper, is a terrible idea in reality. There's nothing sexy about a yeast infection.

ANGELINE, 38
Elkhart, Indiana

Because women wear so many hats, there's a part of us that wouldn't mind someone else taking control for a little bit, so we don't have to make the decisions. When I was married, so much of the decision making was left to me, and there was a certain point when I was like, "Please, somebody make the decisions besides me!" If this puts women in that frame of mind, more power to them.

AMANDA, 31
VALPARAISO, IN

I WAS EXTREMELY SHY WITH TALKING TO MY HUSBAND ABOUT MY FANTASIES AND WHAT I WANTED SEXUALLY. AFTER READING THE BOOK, I AM MUCH MORE CONFIDENT WHEN TALKING TO MY HUSBAND AND NOT SO SHY WHEN IT COMES TO WHAT I WANT.

> I THINK WOMEN LIKE TO BE DOMINATED. I THINK WHETHER OR NOT WE WANT TO ADMIT IT, WE WANT THE DOMINANT GUY BECAUSE IT MAKES US FEEL DESIRED AND COVETED.
> LYNDSY, 32
> MARINA DEL REY, FL

WHY SHOULD YOU HAVE BEEN CAST AS ANASTASIA STEELE?

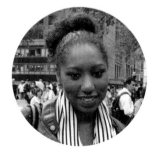

Nicole, Brooklyn, NY
"She's argumentative and keeps Christian on his toes, and I do the same."

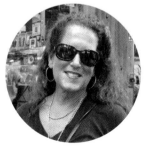

Terry, Palm Beach, FL
"I'm very conservative, and I tend to gravitate toward controlling men."

I THINK MY HUSBAND, LIKE MANY BRITISH MEN, WOULD BE TERRIFIED IF I SUDDENLY INTRODUCED DUCT TAPE, TIE WRAPS AND ROPE INTO THE BEDROOM. HE'D PROBABLY WONDER IF I WAS MENOPAUSAL!

SALLY, 49
DERBYSHIRE, BRITAIN

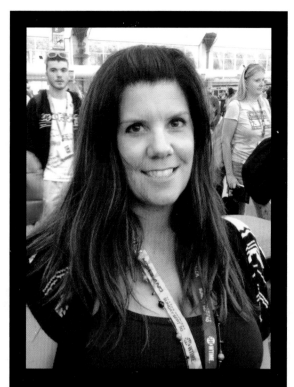

HOLLY, 40
Irvine, CA

So you've never had sex before, you meet a guy and he's like, "Welcome to my playroom..." What do you do? I'd be running the other way! I might go just out of curiosity to see what it's all about. I probably would at least go, but I don't know. When the contract showed up I was like, "Holy cow!" I was shocked at how spelled out everything was. It was very specific. That's a big time warning.

JAYME, 39
IRVINE, CA

My 65-year-old mother turned me on to it. It's the only book she's recommended I read. I'd just finished reading The Hunger Games so...I was looking for a new book, and she suggested Fifty Shades of Grey. I could see why she was into it! When she recommended it, she said, "Get to chapter six and you'll be hooked."

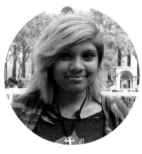

Devika, Guyana
"I love bondage. I really do, all the handcuffs and the whips."

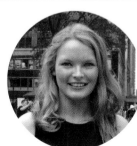

Olivia, Birmingham, UK
"I want to marry Mr. Grey. Period."

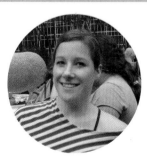

Annabelle, New York, NY
"I would be the worst Ana. I lost my virginity when I was 18."

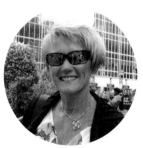

Barbara, Gainesville, FL
"I wouldn't. I'd be too paranoid about the guy just being a total nut."

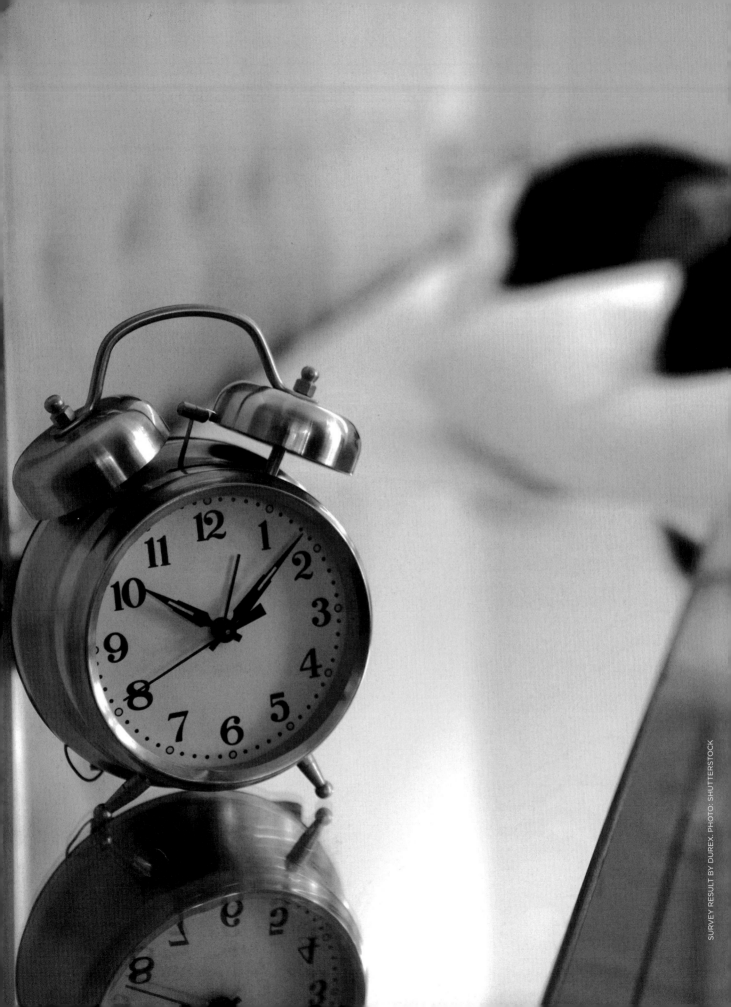

1 in 4 adults said they prefer their lovemaking last 10 minutes or less.

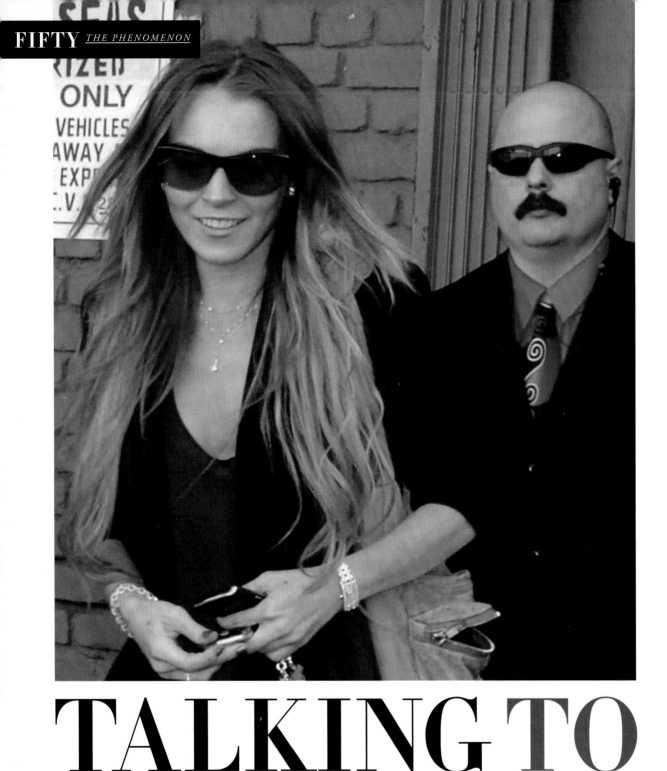

TALKING TO TAYLOR

Celebrity bodyguard Kris Herzog (above, right, with Lindsay Lohan) reveals what it's like to be a real-life security guard and confidant for high-profile clients.

Most of your team is made up of former Navy SEALs and other elite members of the Armed forces. What's more difficult, taking out a target like Osama bin Laden or protecting a strong-willed client like Lindsay Lohan?

When you're a member of the Delta Force and you're going to get bin Laden, you have the complete support of the U.S. government watching your back. As a celebrity bodyguard, it's exactly the opposite. You have the support of no one, and if you screw up, you are going to be disavowed immediately. You'll be criminally tried and civilly sued.

Christian and Taylor are seemingly always close to one another. Do you tune out clients' private conversations or do you listen in and chuckle?

If it's a client I have a strong personal relationship with, not only do I listen, I take notes, because eight hours later they may turn and say, "What time am I supposed to be there to have dinner again?"

Where do you draw the line on who you'd take a bullet for?

I live by a sense of honor, duty, country and self. I would step between any client and a bullet because I won't take on a client I don't respect. In *Fifty Shades*, Christian recognizes Taylor is probably the only person who might step between him and a bullet. Usually you become friends and the client trusts you with their life, and, in exchange, you receive great compensation and long-term job security.

What's the protocol when your client decides they want to get frisky in the back seat while you're on duty?

If it's a male client you make sure it's consensual, make sure you're not being set up for a blackmail scheme. If it's a female client, you make sure she isn't drunk or under the influence and has her wits about her to make an informed decision. And you make sure you can always hear her so that if she calls for help, you can rush into the room and save her life.

The Navy SEAL Bodyguard Group and
The Bodyguard Group of Beverly Hills, est. 1967.
See their 47-year history in photos and videos at
TheBodyguardGroup.com; KrisHerzog.com

POCKET PROTECTOR

Five things Kris Herzog, and probably Taylor, never leave home without.

CONDOMS
"There are many times you are there to protect the client from themselves."

SWALLOWABLE GPS DEVICES
"If we were kidnapped and realized we were at a point of no return, we could both swallow these. They could strip us naked, but we still could be secretly tracked by GPS."

DISGUISED CANS OF PEPPER SPRAY
"It might look like a cigarette lighter, a ballpoint pen or a cellphone, but it's actually pepper spray that shoots 20 feet."

TASER GUN
"Three-shot taser, each shot can go 35 feet."

BREATH FRESHENER & MOUTHWASH
"Even A-List celebrities are plagued by bad breath."

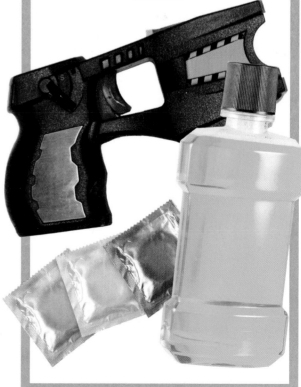

10

THINGS I
LEARNED
ABOUT DATING
A MILLIONAIRE

y-five-year-old Claire Paul looked to *seekingarrangement.com* and

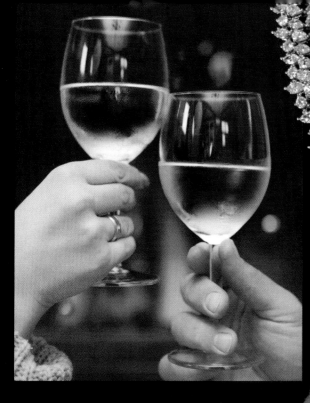

1 **You never have to worry about anything.**
He pays people to take care of all the trivial details of his life so we can enjoy each other effortlessly.

2 **The difference isn't just the money.**
It's the types of things you do and his attitude. He's completely sure of himself and gets away with things other people don't.

3 **You're gifted over-the-top luxuries.**
He bought me a Cartier watch that was probably about $15,000.

4 **You eat extravagant meals.**
We flew to the French Laundry, near Napa, randomly for his friend's vineyard opening.

5 **Men with money need someone adventurous in the bedroom.**
They bore easily and need you to keep them on their toes. My Sugar Daddy's not controlling, though.

6 **You have a comfortable outlet to experiment in the bedroom.**
Ana sometimes seems a bit naïve. I'm very open sexually, and that's one of the things my Sugar Daddy loves about me. Once, we were in Vegas for the weekend and spent thousands of dollars on sex toys for the penthouse suite. Then we just left it all in the room when we checked out. I can't imagine what the maids thought.

7 **He has the tact and power to express himself sexually.**
It comes naturally to a powerful and strategic businessman.

8 **Don't wait around for something like this to happen to you.**
I wanted the relationship just as badly as he did, and that's why I went on *seekingarrangement.com* in the first place, which is where I met him.

9 **You discover you have expensive taste in all facets of life.**
I love oysters. He doesn't like them, so I get to eat them all, which I prefer.

10 **Things can get out of hand.**
We've been to Miami and Vegas and gone on crazy shopping trips. He bought me a Chanel purse in Vegas and offered to pay for a car, but I don't want that. If we ever had a falling out, I would feel weird driving it.

Men are much more likely than women—48% vs. 28%—to fall in love at first sight.

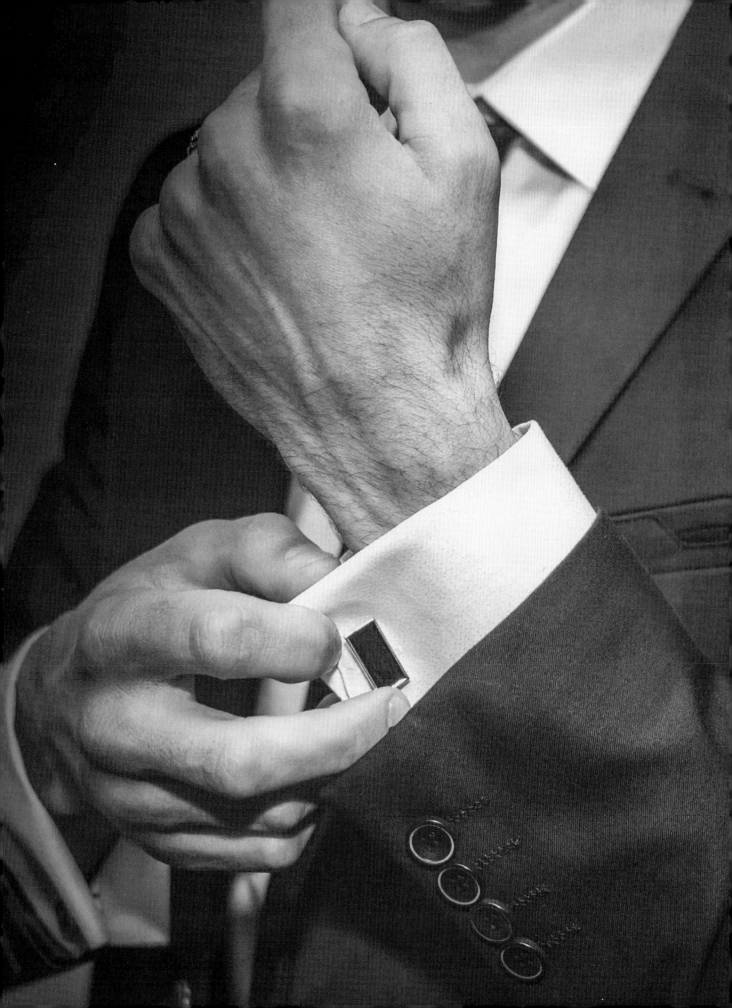

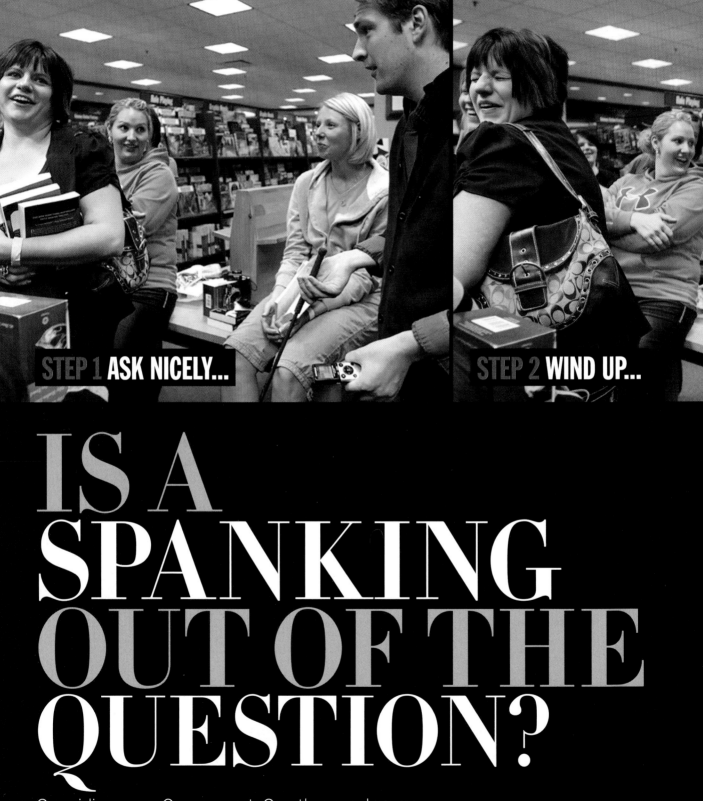

STEP 1 ASK NICELY...

STEP 2 WIND UP...

IS A SPANKING OUT OF THE QUESTION?

One riding crop. One request. One thousand women.
How would you react to this painful focus group?

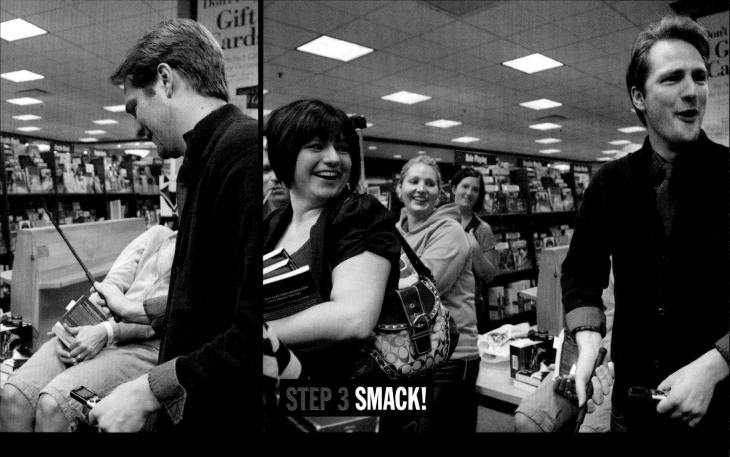

STEP 3 **SMACK!**

THE QUEST AND QUESTION

If a stranger approached you with very little pretense and produced a riding crop, then asked if he could spank you, how would you react? What if he said please? Would you laugh in his face, call the cops, or would you dutifully bend over? Would your answer change if you were surrounded by a group of your peers waiting in line to get E L James's autograph?

I thought I knew the answers to these questions even though I've never pretended to know everything about women. In fact, when I claim to know anything about women, I'm probably pretending. But one thing I can say definitively, because the numbers back me up, is that a lot of women love *Fifty Shades of Grey*. I know some love the romance, some love the sex and some love both. Some call it a guilty pleasure, others guiltlessly find pleasurable passages on every page. Whatever their reasons for reading it, all of them love Christian Grey.

I'm a lot of things, but Christian Grey I am not. I'm a little older, a lot poorer and I've never been in a helicopter. I own exactly seven ties.

But I felt of all the things Christian Grey is (a billionaire CEO, master of all things sexual, really good at wearing pants) the easiest thing to imitate would be his penchant for punishment in the bedroom. Anyone can give a spanking, right? There was just one problem: I had no idea if that was a part of his personality women found appealing. I wanted to know if women only enjoy reading about being spanked or if a nice, hard swat was something many of them secretly—or openly—craved.

I flew across the country to Minneapolis, Minnesota, where E L James was scheduled to do a signing at a local Barnes & Noble. When I arrived at the bookstore, fresh off a plane from New York, I immediately realized I was out of my depth. There were nearly 1,000 women (and a few men) lined up in the store, some of whom had arrived the night before and camped out on the sidewalk. None of them were wearing signs that said, "Yes, reporter from New York, I would like a spanking," which meant I was going to have to start asking around.

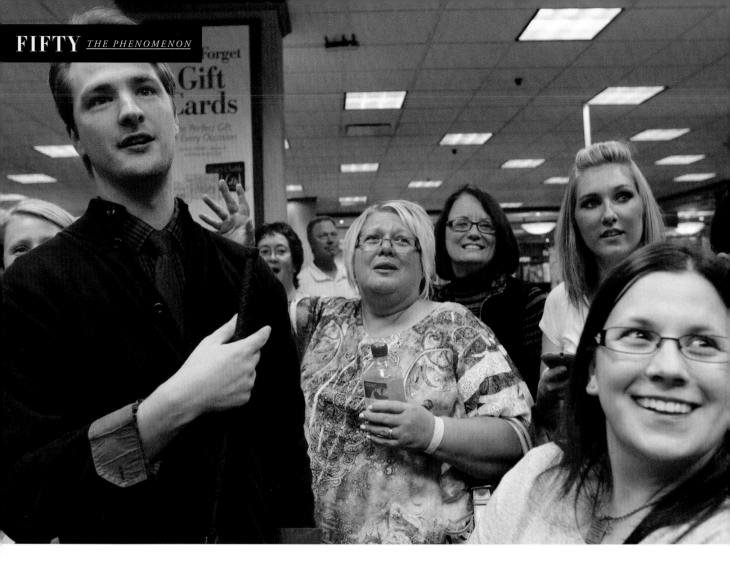

"EVER SEEN ONE OF THESE?"

"Have you ever seen one of these before?" I asked, pulling a black, leather-tipped riding crop out of my bag, presenting it like Excalibur. Two young women in their early 20s stepped forward instantly. I asked them a few simple, fairly standard queries such as, "What do you like most about Christian Grey?" and, "Would you ever sign a sex contract?" It was a casual conversation with very low stakes. When both women agreed they would sign a contract "if it was Christian Grey's," I decided it was time for my follow-up. "So...can I spank you with this?" I asked, doing my best to maintain my journalistic integrity without sounding like some kind of late-night Cinemax cliché.

And that's when the world slowed down. A large crowd of women began to gather around to listen in on our conversation. A slow gasp erupted into a chorus of "Oh my God" 's and "holy crap" 's. I had their full attention. "Where?" one smiled.

"Anywhere. You pick," I said, more nervous than she was. I explained that if she let me spank her, she'd be allowed to hit me in kind, as hard as she pleased. This seemed to be the sweetener she needed. We settled on the underside of her forearm. I tapped her lightly and she gasped, probably at how tame the whole thing was.

"Now it's your turn," she laughed. She enthusiastically swatted me on the rear, and the crowd of women cheered at our little show. I felt like *Magic Mike*'s slightly masochistic and uncoordinated stepbrother. And that's when things started to heat up.

PACK LEADER

Emboldened by the cheers (and the smack on the butt) I opened up the question to the floor. "Who wants a spanking?" I bellowed, though a far-off observer might have assumed I was doing my best *Gladiator* impression, asking the gathering crowd whether or not they were entertained. I made a slow turn, taking them all

"These were leaders of the PTA, small business owners, mothers of five; and all of them were making me feel sexually inadequate."

in, and raised the riding crop into the air like the leader of a jockey revolution. I was shocked at the show of hands. Nearly every woman within earshot was interested in a playful swat. A woman of about 30 insisted she be next and made no secret about where she wanted the blow to land. "Right on the butt," she laughed as everyone applauded. I flicked the riding crop forward.

"That's all you've got?" she asked. I felt even less like Mr. Grey than when I'd started. "I just didn't want to hurt you...." I muttered. We hadn't even agreed on a safe word.

Someone over my shoulder quipped that a little pain was the point. "You want me to go again?" I asked, wishing I'd stuck with those tennis lessons my parents had sprung for in 8th grade.

She wiggled her rump as a response. These women were all rooting for me to swing a riding crop at a stranger as hard as I could. One of them questioned my masculinity. Another asked if I'd ever done this before. I thought at any moment they might pounce, using their collection of souvenir grey ties to bind me and show me how it was done. These were leaders of the PTA, small business owners, mothers of five; and all of them were making me feel sexually inadequate. It was as though I was being bullied into being a bully. I cocked my arm and zeroed in. I imagined a horsefly, the same one that killed my family and flew off with our life savings, had landed on her backside. I was the only one who could stop it from killing again, but I had to be swift, direct, unmerciful. I whipped the riding crop through the air and it whistled for a split second before landing with a crack against her denim-clad derrière.

Her tepid reaction led me to believe she was keeping her copy of *Fifty* in her back pocket. "My turn," she snapped over her shoulder, a devilish look in her eye. The crowd simultaneously said, "Ooooooo" the way a sitcom audience does when the wacky neighbor accidentally breaks the urn containing grandma's ashes. I was worried. These women were out for blood. They weren't like Ana at all. They were all secretly just like Christian, and every one of them wanted nothing more than to exercise some inner demons by smacking my rear. I was in deep, deep trouble.

And then, either because the group was being too loud, or because it was apparent my screams were about to be, the cops crashed the party.

AN ELEMENT OF DANGER

"That's a weapon," said Officer Buzzkill. (Editor's note: this was not his real name.) "A weapon?" I asked, incredulous. I knew from experience the good people of the TSA did not consider the riding crop to be a threat (see page 116), and I didn't see much reason for security at Barnes & Noble to be tighter than what you'd find while trying to board a plane. Still, arguing with a uniformed police officer 1,000 miles away from my home (and my lawyer) seemed like a bad idea.

"It's a weapon. You can do that off the property but not here," he stated flatly. The women booed. I explained to the officer that I had no idea a riding crop was a weapon. He said he'd hang on to it until after the event. I quietly handed it over. The woman who owed me a spanking was not pleased, and she raised her hand as if saying, "We're not finished here."

As the officer walked away, I quietly produced a flogger from my bag, earning points for showing a crowd of women a toy that until that evening many of them had only read about. I was Prometheus

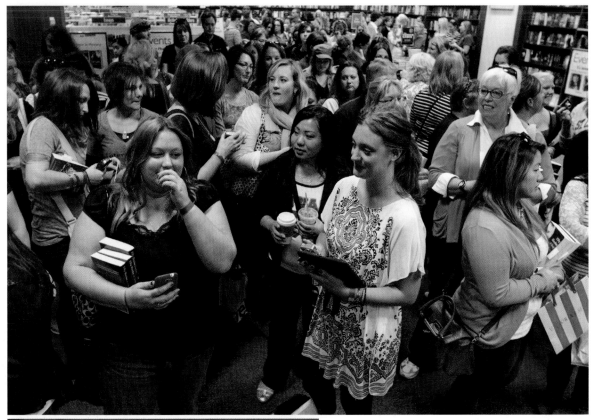

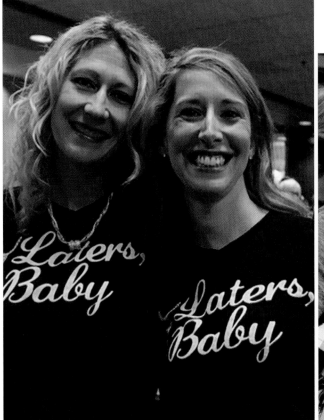

Laters, Baby The women waiting in line to meet E L James were from all walks of life, but they all had one thing in common: a love of *Fifty Shades of Grey*.

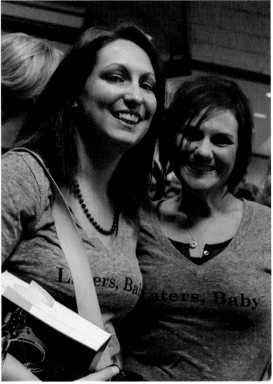

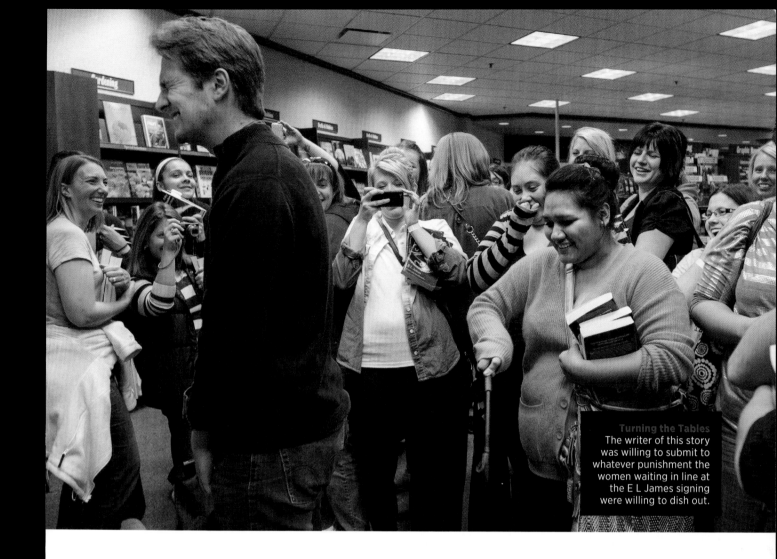

(the Firebringer, not the *Alien* non-prequel), and I'd opened their eyes. I went from being "the guy with the riding crop" to being "the guy who loves *Fifty Shades* more than we do." One woman invited me to her *Fifty Shades* theme party. Others asked if I would pose for pictures. I even signed some of their bras.

THE REAL STAR

But my fame was short-lived. While I previously felt I held these women in the palm of my hand, I realized rather quickly that the only reason they were transfixed by me was because I was a passing stand-in for a character created by their real hero. These women didn't want a spanking from me; they wanted one from Christian Grey. But they all wanted one, and sometimes you take what you can get. Still, when E L James entered the bookstore, she was welcomed with a roar reserved for royalty—or at least the Kings of Leon. They greeted James like a rockstar because she'd changed their lives in ways even the greatest songs can't compete with. E L James knows more

about women than I ever will. She knows what they desire, what they hold dear and what they think about the choice between reality and fantasy: They don't want to choose. They simultaneously seek safety and danger, security and uncertainty. They want to read the book and see the movie.

E L James signed books for three hours. She cracked jokes. She posed for photos. She flirted with the police officer standing next to her after noticing his belt had a set of silver handcuffs and in his cargo pants pocket was a black riding crop; he quickly became the talk of the line. I laughed to myself. While he'd prevented me from discovering just how many women in the crowd would let me spank them, he'd also taught me something: You can turn a lot of women's heads by pulling a riding crop out of a bag and asking, "Can I spank you?" But you'll make a stronger impression by standing quietly, implement of pain displayed subtly at your side, leading women of all ages to quietly approach you, knowing smiles under sideways glances to ask, "Will you spank me with that?" It's the main reason I asked for it back.

INSIDE THE MALE MIND

Statistics, candid quotes and one fireman's testimony offer a look at what guys really think about your recent obsession.

Firemen are right at home with a little heat, which is one reason Brendan Montgomery, a fireman from Louisville, Kentucky, read the steamy *Fifty* novels.

Why *Fifty Shades of Grey*?
I was at the firehouse, and we were watching the news in the morning, and I saw that some people were upset about it. And I was looking through my Nook library, and one of my cousins had downloaded the books. So I thought, "I'll find out for myself what I think about it."

Did you read it in the firehouse?
I do almost all my reading there because, when you have a 16-month-old at home, it's actually quieter. A couple of us have been reading it, but nobody's going to admit it. I know they've read it, because they've made a few comments that you would have had to read the book to know about.

What does your wife think about *Fifty Shades*?
My wife hasn't read it. I felt like I couldn't tell her what I was reading until I was done. She thought I was reading a book about Steve Jobs. She was a bit surprised when she found out. I still want her to read it.

Tell us the truth: Did you enjoy it?
It's kind of a romantic comedy. The email conversations in the book had me laughing out loud. It's not supposed to be an action movie. He's always doing something wrong, or she's always doing something wrong. I mean, you have to read 150 pages before you get to the first sex scene.

What do you think is the most unrealistic thing about Christian Grey?
The most honest answer? That he can have sex, then turn around and have sex five minutes later.

HERE'S WHAT I LEARNED: IF I'M LUCKY, I'LL ONE DAY BE AS RICH AS THAT GUY. IN THE MEANTIME, I CAN BE MORE ATTENTIVE TO MY WIFE. THAT'S FREE.
MAX, 31 // STAMFORD, CONNECTICUT

Did you openly read *Fifty Shades* in public?

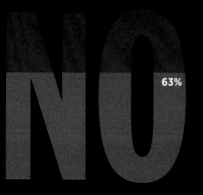

NO
63%

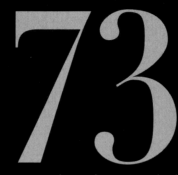

73

Percentage of men who would prefer the female first broach the subject of role-play, for fear of giving the impression they are bored with their sex lives.

The order of importance to men when introducing erotica into the bedroom.

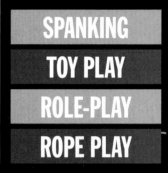

SPANKING

TOY PLAY

ROLE-PLAY

ROPE PLAY

Which woman from *Fifty Shades* would you most want to date?

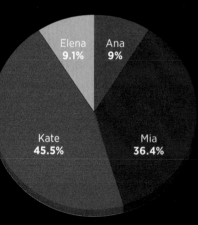

Elena 9.1%
Ana 9%
Kate 45.5%
Mia 36.4%

I LEARNED TO WASH MY HANDS EACH TIME I USE AN ELEVATOR.
REX, 29 // LOS ANGELES, CALIFORNIA

If men could change one thing about their sex lives, increasing the duration in which they engage in the act (average is 3-10 minutes) tops the list.

IF THIS IS WHAT WOMEN TRULY WANT, I HAVE A LOT OF WORK TO DO. STEP ONE: BUY SEXIER PANTS.
JEFF, 36 // CHARLOTTE, NORTH CAROLINA

3% OF MEN HAVE NEVER HEARD OF *FIFTY SHADES OF GREY*.

I PROMISED MY WIFE I'D BE A BETTER LOVER IF SHE PROMISED NEVER TO MENTION THE NAME "CHARLIE TANGO" EVER AGAIN. DAVE, 38 //
SEASIDE HEIGHTS, NEW JERSEY

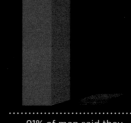

91% of men said they would gladly read erotica with their partners, if they in turn agreed to watch pornography with them.

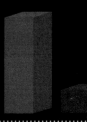

81% of men think *Fifty Shades* has helped their partners become more expressive when discussing sexuality.

35% of men get aroused by *steamy kisses.*

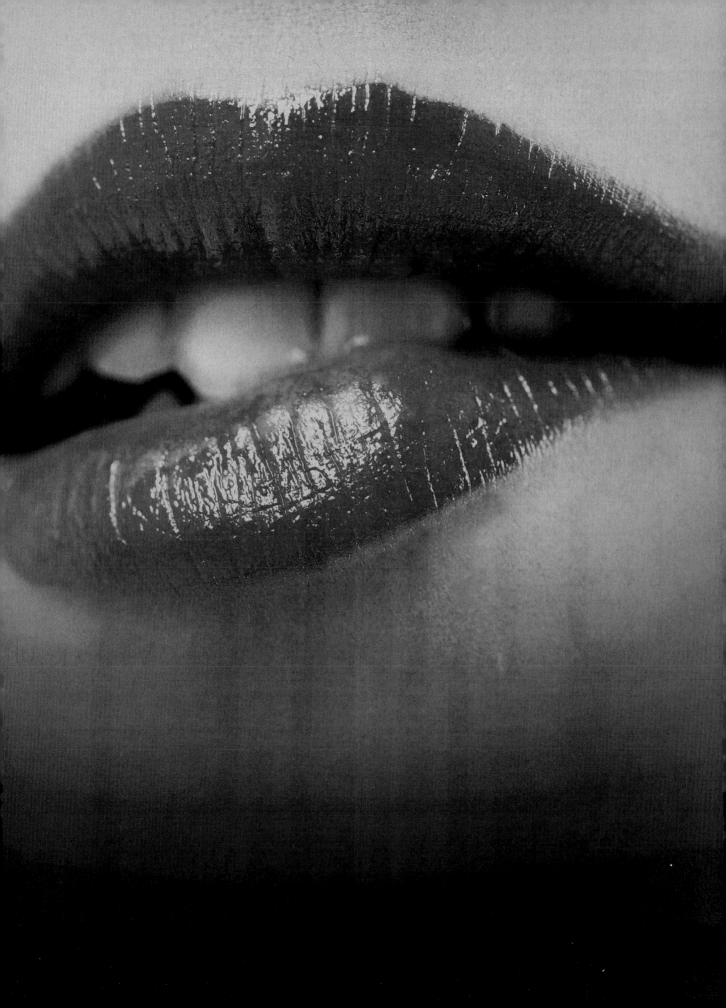

74% OF MEN SURVEYED FEEL THEY ARE LESS EXPRESSIVE THAN THEIR FEMALE COUNTERPARTS

W

"e have a new patient," Dr. B. announced. "James. He's young. He seems sweet. Pretty nervous, though. Be gentle with him. He'll be right in." She handed me his file. I smiled, looking over his forms, knowing I'd soon be getting to know this guy very well.

When a patient came for his first appointment with the doctor, she'd go over various aspects of sexual history with him—the age he first had sex, how many partners, how often with and without a partner. Her professional, yet warm, demeanor, coupled with all the degrees and accolades that lined the walls of her office, made patients feel comfortable sharing such intimate information. That, or their desire to truly be cured of whatever problem had brought them here in the first place.

The doctor and I treated a host of issues: erectile dysfunction, premature or delayed ejaculation, inability to touch or be touched, even removing fixations with particular fetishes if a patient found them impeding his personal life. In my time working with her, all of our patients were male. And many sought treatment to improve an existing sexual relationship, whether within a long-term marriage or with a girlfriend. Some patients were shy or socially awkward; others were outgoing and seemed confident. All were generally successful at work. Age, nationality and physical type varied greatly among patients—the oldest I worked with was in his 70s, and the youngest was 21 and still in college. I was just shy of 30. An initial program of treatment was six two-hour sessions a week at our office, with the session's first half consisting of traditional talk therapy with Dr. B, and the second, a series of exercises that took place with me in my private room.

As I waited for my part of the session to begin with James, I readied my room, straightening the couch pillows, putting on quiet music (I often preferred playing Billie Holiday or Nina Simone), generally making things seem comfortable for someone who might be jumpy. According to what the doctor had gleaned, James was uncomfortable with being touched even though he was in a relationship—an obvious obstacle to intimacy. There was a knock at the door, and the doctor ushered in a handsome, well-dressed, definitely young-looking man. I rose to shake his hand. "It's great to meet you," I welcomed him. "Have a seat right here." I indicated a spot next to where I'd sit on the couch. After some small talk about where he worked and the weather in Chicago (yes, the weather), I asked James some direct questions about what

"I truly felt I was helping these men. And in actuality, I was also helping women."

I'd learned from his file. How exactly was he uncomfortable being touched? According to him, he was able to have intercourse with the woman he had been dating (and, prior to her, two others), but only quickly, in the dark, with his eyes closed. Other kinds of direct stimulation, he explained, felt good initially, but failed to make him aroused. A woman's touch felt too light, like a tickling sensation, more a "funny" feeling rather than a good one. Still, he was really into his lady-friend and wanted to have better sex with her. I'd dealt with similar situations, men with difficulty getting physically turned on despite a desire to do so. For the remainder of our first hour together, I tried to make James as comfortable as I could. I sensed a lot of nervousness from him in his tense body language and lack of eye contact.

I massaged his hands with increasing amounts of pressure to see what felt good to him. I encouraged him to do the same to me. By the end of the session he seemed more relaxed,

but we had a long way to go. Our sessions progressed. We had some success with games and role-playing scenarios regarding relaxation and touch. Eventually I asked James to undress, and he did, with some hesitation. I did the same (I liked to wear wrap dresses to work. Easy on, easy off!). "I know you're not good with being touched," I began, "so this might help you feel more in control." After some breathing exercises, I had James take my hand and guide it all over his body as if they were his own, starting from the neck area, heading downward, slowly, without rushing to the genital area. "You can close your eyes if this is embarrassing," I suggested, but he kept them open, explaining this helped him feel even more sure of what was happening. After a number of minutes of running my hand, controlled by his, over his chest and legs, he stopped.

"It's OK, let's do this together," I said.

"I feel like I'm cheating on my girlfriend,"

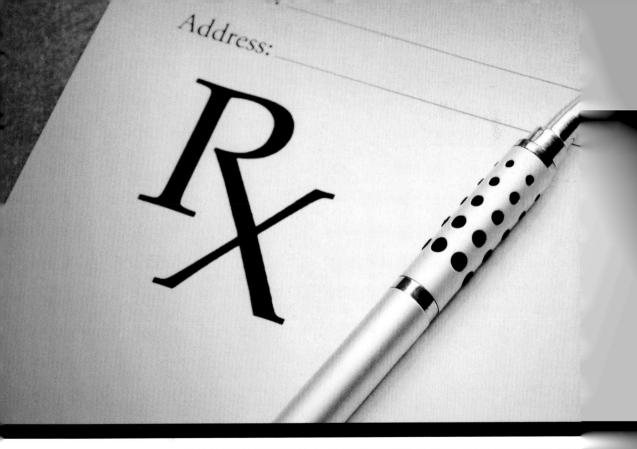

IT'S ESTIMATED THAT 20 MILLION MEN IN THE U.S. SUFFER FROM SEXUAL DYSFUNCTION ISSU

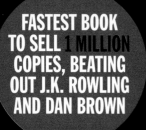

FASTEST BOOK TO SELL 1 MILLION COPIES, BEATING OUT J.K. ROWLING AND DAN BROWN

A FAMILY AFFAIR

Two generations of women come together around one seminal read.

The *Fifty Shades* trilogy has created nothing short of a whirlwind; mothers, daughters and even grandmothers have explored its pages, and as a result, they're now more comfortable exploring the subject of sex with one another. What started out as whispered gossip over the back fence has turned into one of the best-selling books in history. *Fifty Shades of Grey* has, without a doubt, tied these women together—no pun intended.

1 Sharon Lippman, 40 // Scarsdale, NY and Sara Handelsman, 66 // Delray, FL

How did you feel about your mom reading *Fifty Shades*?

Sharon I couldn't wait for her to read it. I've always gotten a kick out of tormenting her about sex. I have no shame and love to make her blush. I knew she'd love *Fifty*. She loves a good love story.

Did you talk about the books after she read them?

Sharon It took her a while to read them after I initially begged her to, but when she finally did, I was thrilled. I told her, "Finally! I'm so proud of

you." She said, somewhat sheepishly, "I read the first one twice." I gave her a big smile and said, "Now I'm really proud of you." That was the extent of our conversation. We had lots of knowing looks, smiles and laughs.

How has your relationship benefited from the books?

Sharon For me, as a mother myself, I've been able to see my mom as a woman in her own right more clearly. So, our shared enjoyment of the *Fifty* trilogy is just one more way in which I've been able to see, and get close to, the real woman underneath my mom.

2 Lisa Shaller-Goldberg, 48 // New York, NY and Arlene Shaller, 71 // Woodland Park, NJ

When did you decide to share the trilogy with your mom?

Lisa My mother was going on vacation, and before I had started to read the book, I had recommended it to her. Once I discovered what it was about, I was a little embarrassed about telling my mom to read it. I called her to tell her I didn't think she would like it and, lo and

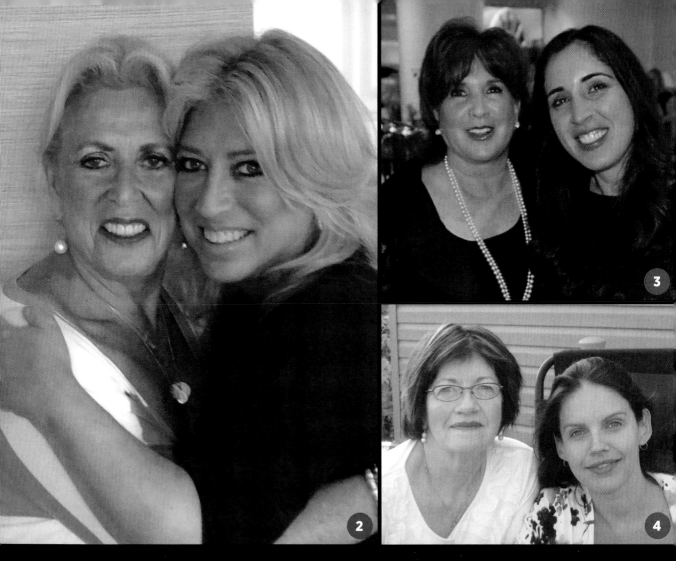

behold, she was deep into the second book and completely obsessing.

Did you have a conversation about the books after they read them?

Lisa Of course. We were obsessed to the point that we were on the search for the real-life Christian Grey.

3 Jaclyn Coleman, 35 and Linda Schnieder, 58 // New York, NY

When did you decide you were going to share the trilogy with your mom?

Jaclyn Pretty soon after I read it, I told my mother about it. I was curious what she was going to think about it. I found out she was actually reading it, too! Her friend had told her about it.

Were you nervous about how she was going to react to the book or to you reading it?

Jaclyn No, we sell vibrators together. No topic is off limits.

What was your mom's reaction to you suggesting the trilogy to her?

Jaclyn She enjoyed reading the books and being part of the whole *Fifty Shades* phenomenon.

4 Michele Ashe, 36 and Linda Zuzanski, 62 // Winnipeg, Manitoba, Canada

Which one of you read *Fifty Shades* first?

Michele My mother. I saw she was reading a book before bed in the hotel while on a family trip, but I only saw the cover. When we came back to Winnipeg, the girls who work at the sex shop my mother owns kept saying, "People were coming in about this book, we have to read it." My mom asked, "What are you talking about?" One of our employees said, "Well, I have at least one person a day come in saying they read this book, *Fifty Shades of Grey*." I looked at my mom and said, "That's what you're reading? I thought i was a book about menopause!"

What's your overall opinion of the book?

Michele I've always liked romance stories, and I've never read anything like it before. I thought it was pretty racy. And I'm pretty sure she loved the books. She read the whole trilogy within a week.

*Compiled by Lyss Stern, founder of DivaLysscious Moms (DivaMoms.com), a luxury lifestyle company for more than 450,000 moms.

Keeping Count
Anastasia rolls her
eyes 14 times and
bites her lip 43 times
in the book. She
knows how much
Christian hates that...

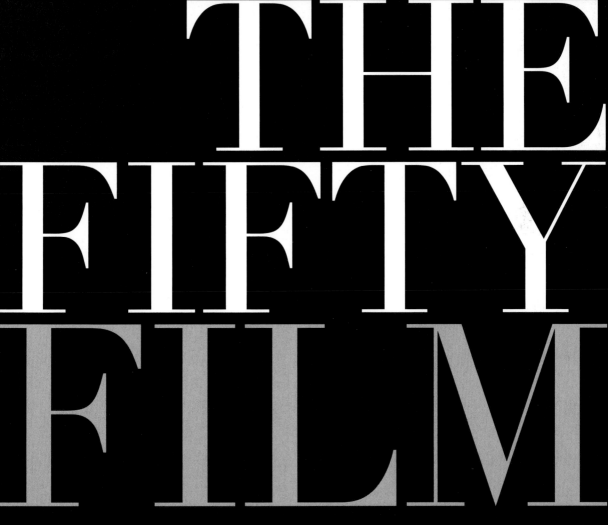

THE FIFTY FILM

Explore the cast, crew and creative minds bringing the erotic story to life.

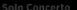

Solo Concerto
Jamie Dornan as Christian and Dakota Johnson as Ana in one of the book's most memorable scenes in which she quietly approaches Christian, who's playing a piece by Alessandro Marcello, following their first night together. After landing the role, Johnson admitted to the *Today* show that she sees a lot of herself in Ana.

CASTING CALL

Choosing the right actors to bring E L James's work to the big screen took all of Hollywood—and most of the Internet.

By the end of 2013, the saga surrounding *Fifty Shades of Grey*'s casting was almost as much a pop-culture lightning rod as the book itself. Since the film version of E L James's phenomenon was announced, fans of the franchise waited with bated breath to see who would be the real-life manifestations of their favorite characters. Tens of thousands even attempted to assert their will over the casting process with petitions and agitation. But the excitement wasn't limited to readers; some of Hollywood's most recognizable names made their interest in the project immediately known. So many names ended up in play for the roles of Christian and Anastasia that casting the film became a remarkable ordeal.

As early as February 2013, *Gossip Girl*'s Chace Crawford publicly stated he'd love to be involved with the film, and though he didn't specifically say he was aiming for the role of Christian Grey, his fans immediately took up the mantle of support. In April, *The Vampire Diaries*' Ian Somerhalder threw his hat into the ring, saying on *On Air With Ryan Seacrest*, "[Being cast] would be an incredible thing. Hopefully that could pan out." By April 17, Somerhalder fans had created a "trailer" for a version of *Fifty Shades* starring Somerhalder and *Gilmore Girls*' Alexis Bledel—the video garnered nearly 1 million views. Soon, *True Blood*'s Alexander Skarsgård was on the air with *Access Hollywood* saying he was "born to play" Christian Grey.

A BRIEF TIMELINE OF *FIFTY*

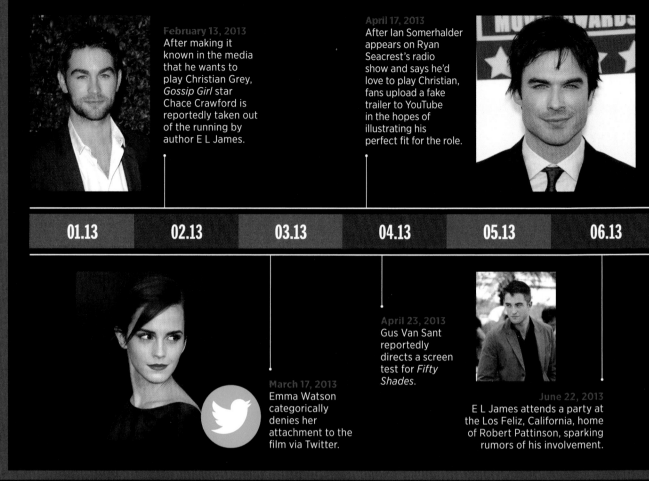

February 13, 2013
After making it known in the media that he wants to play Christian Grey, *Gossip Girl* star Chace Crawford is reportedly taken out of the running by author E L James.

April 17, 2013
After Ian Somerhalder appears on Ryan Seacrest's radio show and says he'd love to play Christian, fans upload a fake trailer to YouTube in the hopes of illustrating his perfect fit for the role.

01.13	02.13	03.13	04.13	05.13	06.13

April 23, 2013
Gus Van Sant reportedly directs a screen test for *Fifty Shades*.

March 17, 2013
Emma Watson categorically denies her attachment to the film via Twitter.

June 22, 2013
E L James attends a party at the Los Feliz, California, home of Robert Pattinson, sparking rumors of his involvement.

The same month, Universal Studios and Focus Features stoked the fire by hiring Academy Award Nominee Gus Van Sant to direct a screen test of the scene where Anastasia loses her virginity to Christian. In the Van Sant scene, Alex Pettyfer of *Magic Mike* reportedly played Christian in an unsuccessful attempt to get the famed director involved on a permanent basis. A-listers Robert Pattinson and Charlie Hunnam were front-runners in the ongoing saga of casting, despite lingering fan support for other candidates. Backing for *White Collar*'s Matt Bomer was so strong—even after Hunnam had been officially cast—that a petition started by fans to cast him garnered almost 100,000 signatures. Though Bomer never actually expressed his interest in the role, he nevertheless publicly voiced his thanks.

"I'm so grateful for the fans and touched," said Bomer, who also gave his support to the film's recently announced stars. "I'm looking forward to seeing the movie with Charlie [Hunnam] and Dakota [Johnson]."

Casting Dakota Johnson—daughter of Don Johnson and Melanie Griffith and best known for minor but scene-stealing roles in *21 Jump Street* and *The Social Network*—as the virginal college student Anastasia Steele was a long process in itself. Despite early rumors that Emma Watson was being considered, Watson tweeted on March 17, 2013 in no uncertain terms that she would not be involved with the project. "Who here actually thinks I would do *50 Shades of Grey* as a movie? Like really. For real. In real life," the *Harry Potter* star wrote. *Pretty Little Liars*

SHADES CASTING RUMORS

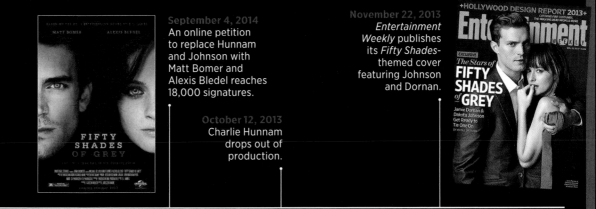

September 4, 2014
An online petition to replace Hunnam and Johnson with Matt Bomer and Alexis Bledel reaches 18,000 signatures.

October 12, 2013
Charlie Hunnam drops out of production.

November 22, 2013
Entertainment Weekly publishes its *Fifty Shades*-themed cover featuring Johnson and Dornan.

07.13	08.13	09.13	10.13	11.13	12.13

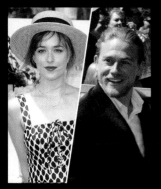

September 2, 2013
E L James announces that Dakota Johnson and Charlie Hunnam have been cast as Christian Grey and Anastasia Steele.

October 23, 2013
Jamie Dornan is announced as the new Christian Grey.

star Lucy Hale auditioned, as did *The Carrie Diaries*' Chloe Bridges, but neither were quite prepared to tackle the subject matter. Hale said the audition made her "uncomfortable," and Bridges didn't mince words with *Cosmopolitan* when asked why she balked at the audition. "The scene was, like, the girl telling her friends about some sexcapade she had," explained Bridges. "But it goes into extreme detail and uses the word 'sperm' a couple times. I was like, 'I don't know, guys, I have to go home to my grandparent's house in a few months at Christmas, I don't know if I can do this.'"

In September 2013, E L James took to Twitter to officially announce Dakota Johnson's casting alongside Charlie Hunnam, and *Fifty Shades*' vocal fandom flooded the Internet with calls

for Hunnam's replacement, which Hunnam seemed to take in stride. However, on October 12, he announced he wouldn't be appearing in the film after all, citing a host of problems, not least of which was the sudden lifestyle change that being involved with a global phenomenon presented. Only 11 days after Hunnam's exit, however, *Once Upon a Time*'s Jamie Dornan was announced as the new Christian Grey. On Thursday, October 24, Dornan's Twitter ballooned to 95,000 followers, and celebrity fans of the books were announcing their newfound love of the Irish actor. By November, the two stars had appeared in character on the cover of *Entertainment Weekly*, and the long, arduous process finally came to an end after one of the most involved castings in movie history.

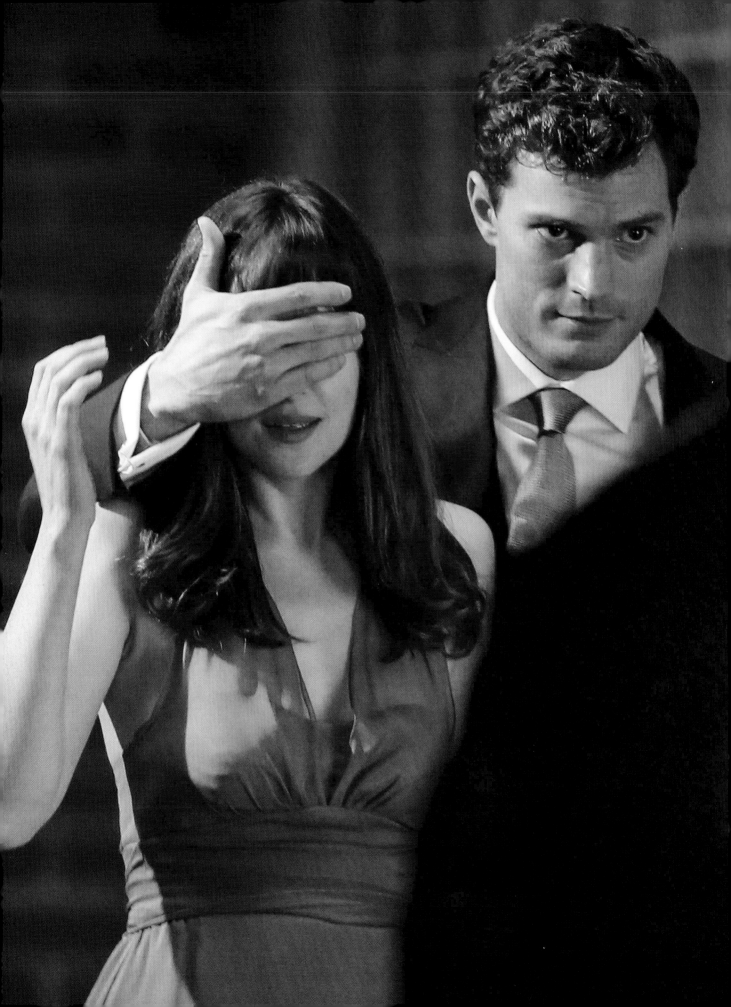

Steamy Sexcapades
Jamie Dornan's Christian Grey
surprises Dakota Johnson's
Anastasia Steele with a $100,000
gift on wheels. The two actors
talked openly on the *Today* show
about filming the book's steamy
sex scenes together, with Johnson
describing them as more of a chore
than a passion-fueled act, while
Dornan added that the scenes were
like "sexual acrobatics."

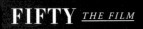

MEET THE CAST

After nearly a year of casting rumors, disapprovals and replacements, the *Fifty* film features talented up-and-comers who will match their faces to the characters beloved by millions of readers.

DAKOTA JOHNSON AS
ANASTASIA STEELE

A rising star signs on for the role of a lifetime.

The only daughter of actors Don Johnson and Melanie Griffith, Dakota Johnson didn't break into Hollywood as much as she grew into it, making her big-screen debut in 1999's *Crazy in Alabama* at just 10 years old. She continued to spend time honing her acting skills and getting accustomed to living under the gaze of the public eye, appearing in a *Teen Vogue* photoshoot alongside other children of celebrities at age 12. After trying her hand at modeling (Johnson appeared in a campaign for Mango Jeans), the actress returned to movies in 2010's *The Social Network* as the eye-catching co-ed who spent a night with Justin Timberlake's Sean Parker. The success of *The Social Network* helped propel Johnson's career, and the actress popped up in Hollywood blockbusters such as *Need for Speed* and *21 Jump Street*, always leaving a favorable impression on audiences. After the cancellation of her short-lived (but critically beloved) sitcom *Ben and Kate*, the 25-year-old actress bounced back by landing the role countless readers had already cast themselves in: Anastasia Steele. Given her history of portraying confident, independent women, there's little doubt her performance in *Fifty Shades of Grey* will leave audiences' palms twitching, ready to applaud.

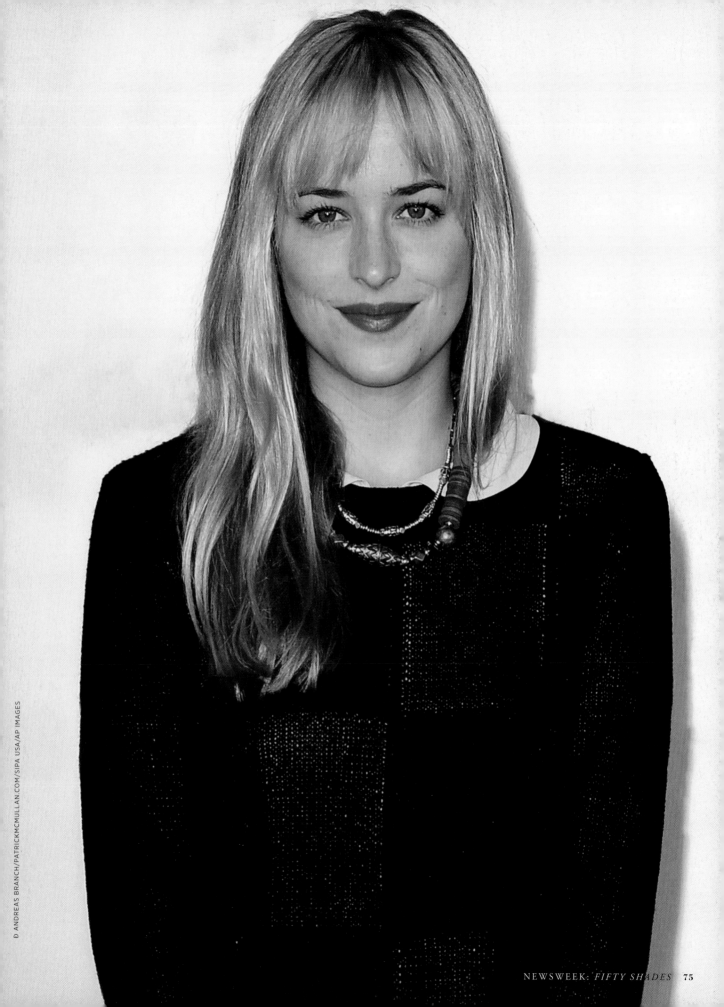

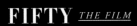

JAMIE DORNAN AS
CHRISTIAN GREY

The Irish actor's past roles speak to his future success as Mr. Grey.

Jamie Dornan's acting resume contains the right mix of sexy and sinister roles to give audiences confidence the 32-year-old actor can pull off playing the controlling lothario. Originally from Belfast in Northern Ireland, Dornan moved to London following his college graduation to pursue his dream of becoming an actor. After seducing Kirsten Dunst's Marie Antoinette as the dashing Count Axel Fersen in Sofia Coppola's stylized biopic, Dornan appeared in several small independent films before breaking out in 2011 as Sheriff Graham/the Huntsman in the ABC television drama *Once Upon a Time*. The role required him to navigate the nuances of playing a justice-obsessed assassin who was also carrying on a secret sexual relationship with the evil mayor.

Dornan's riveting performance in the 2013 British TV series *The Fall* gave the actor a venue to showcase his dark side, portraying a manipulative serial killer who forces his victims to play out his sadistic sexual fantasies. His biggest challenge for the *Fifty* film, though, will be channeling this signature intensity and carnal energy into the role of Christian Grey while maintaining a sympathetic demeanor for audiences. Dornan's good looks (having modeled for Calvin Klein, HUGO and Banana Republic, to name a few) should help take the sting out of his slaps and convince audiences Christian is worth all the baggage—and bondage—he carries with him.

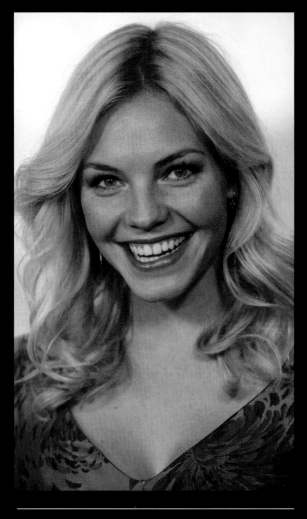

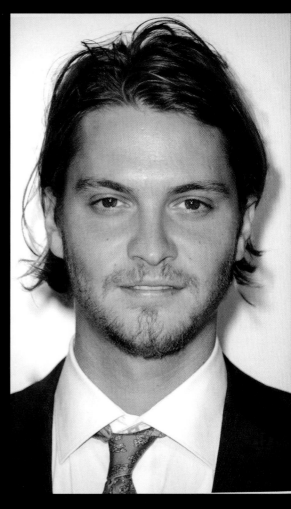

ELOISE MUMFORD AS
KATE KAVANAGH

The stunning Eloise Mumford will portray Anastasia's best friend and roommate, Kate Kavanagh. A graduate of NYU's Tisch School of the Arts, her most memorable roles include Lena Landry on ABC's 2012 horror series *The River* and Lindsay Holloway on the Fox drama *Lone Star*. Her solid performances mark her as perfect to play Kavanagh, a tenacious aspiring journalist. Kate's self-assured poise makes her the polar opposite of Ana, but in spite of their differences, the two remain close throughout the series.

LUKE GRIMES AS
ELLIOT GREY

Known for his roles in the television series *Brothers & Sisters* and *True Blood*, Grimes will continue to charm as Christian Grey's older brother, Elliot. Laid back with a fine sense of humor, Elliot frequently teases his brother, although he proves to be supportive and accompanies Christian to rescue an inebriated Anastasia from a bar. It's there he meets Kate Kavanagh, and the two form an instant attraction that plays out through the rest of the trilogy.

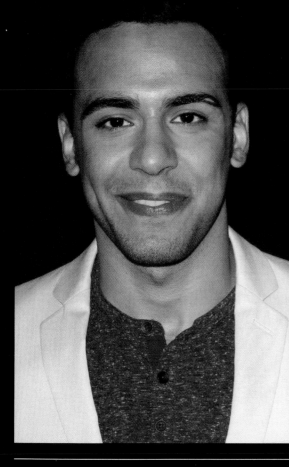

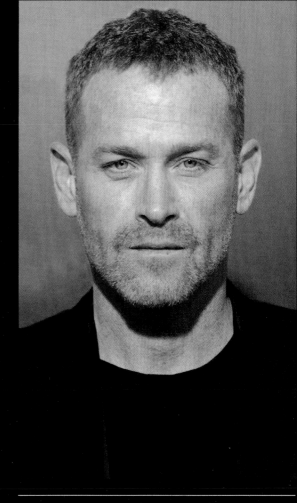

VICTOR RASUK AS
JOSÉ RODRIGUEZ

The star of the HBO series *How to Make It in America* will portray Ana's close friend and photographer, José Rodriguez. José carries a torch for Ana, making him a threat to Christian despite Ana's assurance that he is firmly in the friend zone. After landing the role, Rasuk's relatives showered him with praise. "My aunt loves all three books and said, 'OMG, you're playing José Rodriguez!'" he told *Variety Latino* in the summer of 2014.

MAX MARTINI AS
JASON TAYLOR

Max Martini will lend his gravitas and authoritative presence to the role of bodyguard Jason Taylor. Martini has appeared in several film and television roles, including Corporal Fred Henderson in *Saving Private Ryan* and Master Sergeant Mack Gerhardt on the CBS military drama *The Unit*. Tall and muscular, Taylor is sure to intimidate anyone who tries to harm Grey, though he proves to be kind and sensitive on more than one occasion.

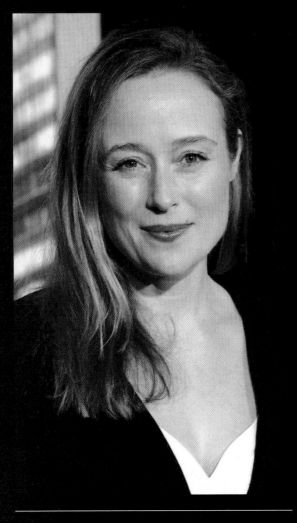

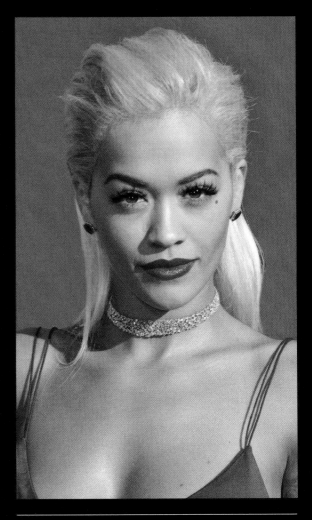

JENNIFER EHLE AS
CARLA MAY WILKS

Most recognized for portraying Elizabeth Bennet in the BBC miniseries *Pride and Prejudice* (and more recently in supporting roles in *The King's Speech* and *Zero Dark Thirty*), Jennifer Ehle will showcase her range by portraying Ana's flighty mother. Characterized by her fleeting hobbies and unsuccessful entrepreneurial schemes, Carla creates tension in her relationship with her daughter.

RITA ORA AS
MIA GREY

Last year, the British singer Rita Ora announced via Twitter she would star as Christian's younger adopted sister, Mia, in the film. This marks Ora's first major movie role, after appearing as a judge on the ninth season of the UK's *X Factor* and as a racer in *Fast & Furious 6*. Though Mia's storyline doesn't take off until the second and third books, we can look to Ora's performance as an indication of what's to come from the *Fifty* franchise.

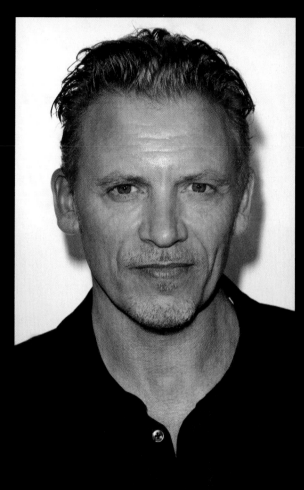

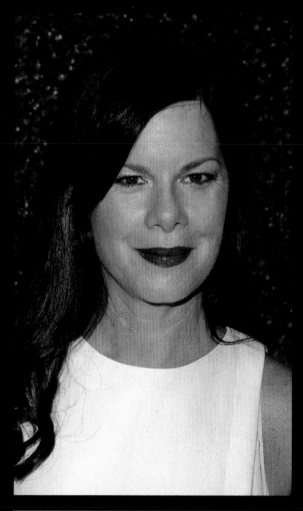

CALLUM KEITH RENNIE AS
RAY STEELE

Canadian character actor Callum Keith Rennie will play Ray Steele, Anastasia's stepfather, whom she considers to be her "real" dad. Rennie's previous roles include Leoben Conoy in *Battlestar Galactica* and Lew Ashby in *Californication*. Ex-military, Steele emphasized the importance of safety and taught Ana self-defense when she was a child. Ray attends Ana's college graduation, where he meets Christian Grey, and the two bond over a shared interest in fly fishing.

MARCIA GAY HARDEN AS
DR. GRACE TREVELYAN GREY

Academy Award winner for her role as Lee Krasner in 2000's *Pollock*, Marcia Gay Harden will star as Dr. Grace Trevelyan Grey, Christian's adoptive mother. She is unaware of her son's previous affair with longtime friend, Elena Lincoln, and expresses delight to find her son with Ana. Harden told *Entertainment Weekly* she doesn't feel fazed by the movie's adult content: "I play Mama Grey, so...unless you're in the red playroom with a toy in your hand and flesh in your face, it's...like any other movie that you could do."

Page Views
Dornan's Mr. Grey pours Johnson's Miss Steele her favorite hot beverage, English breafast tea. The first trailer for *Fifty Shades* garnered more than 36 million views in one week following its premiere on July 24, making it one of the most viewed trailers of 2014.

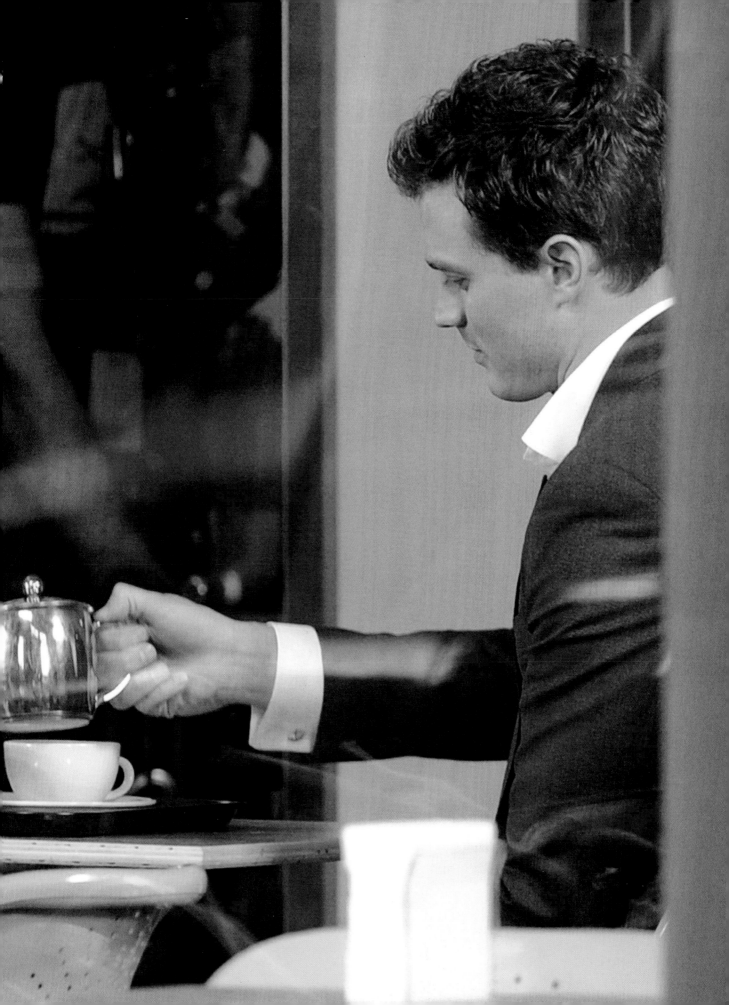

CREATING A SEXUAL STATEMENT

As the intrepid leader of *Fifty Shades*' big-screen makeover,
Sam Taylor-Johnson, a veteran visual artist, is responsible for one of
the most anticipated adaptations in Hollywood history.

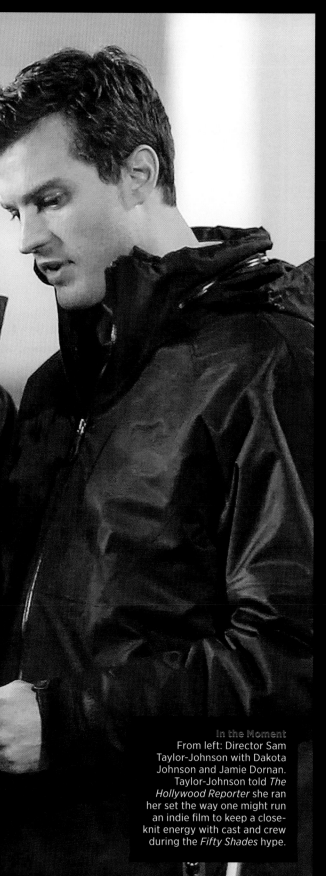

In the Moment
From left: Director Sam Taylor-Johnson with Dakota Johnson and Jamie Dornan. Taylor-Johnson told *The Hollywood Reporter* she ran her set the way one might run an indie film to keep a close-knit energy with cast and crew during the *Fifty Shades* hype.

Even though she's been tasked with directing the first cinematic installment of the most pervasive literary phenomenon of the decade, Sam Taylor-Johnson made it clear early in her tenure that she wasn't stuck on the size of the undertaking. "Those are the questions I find difficult to answer," she told *Harper's Bazaar* in October when asked why the story of Christian and Anastasia is so popular. "I guess I just love the fact that I've never really seen a movie that tackles this subject matter. But from the perspective of the millions of other readers, who knows what it is? It's definitely resonated, that's for sure." Taylor-Johnson was a surprising choice from a field of seasoned directors like Gus Van Sant, but her previous work sheds light on E L James's and Universal's choice.

Taylor-Johnson, née Taylor-Wood, got her start in visual arts before making the transition to film with 2008's *Love You More*—a short-subject in which two young lovers are drawn together by a Buzzcocks song. A video piece of hers showcasing a sleeping David Beckham is featured at London's National Portrait Gallery, and her 2009 John Lennon biopic *Nowhere Boy* showcased her ability to capture a larger-than-life persona accurately and provocatively on screen. After a three-year break from show business during which she married *Nowhere Boy*'s Aaron Taylor-Johnson— né plain old Johnson—and focused on her family, Taylor-Johnson was announced in June 2013 as the woman who would bring *Fifty Shades of Grey* to life.

In addition to her work in cinema, Taylor-Johnson also continues to publish photography. Her 2014 monograph *Second Floor* captures the private apartments of Coco Chanel above her Paris headquarters, and her 18 other publications show the sort of manipulation of imagery and situations that reveal intense psychological conflict—exactly the kind of emotional portraits she's sure to have created for *Fifty Shades of Grey*. A story that has generated debate over whether it's empowering or demeaning toward women, *Fifty Shades* is fortunate to have an experienced female artist deftly handling its on-screen evolution. In a statement released after her announcement as director, Taylor-Johnson said, "For the legions of fans, I want to say that I will honor the power of Erika's book and the characters of Christian and Anastasia. They are under my skin too." But at the same time, Taylor-Johnson, a two-time cancer survivor, has made it clear that she never intended to hold back in her adaptation. "[Surviving cancer] does give you a remarkable perspective on life," she told *Harper's Bazaar* in 2010. "You take no prisoners and just do what feels right in your life."

Taking Stride
On set outside the Grey Enterprises Holdings building, director Sam Taylor-Johnson talks Dornan and Johnson through a scene. Dornan admitted on the UK's "Graham Norton Show" in March that he had to learn how to walk from scratch for his role in the film, to go "heel to toe" instead of his usual "toe to, like, more toe," as he explained.

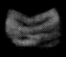

THE NEXT FIFTY

A collection of seductive reads for any fan of E L James's debut.

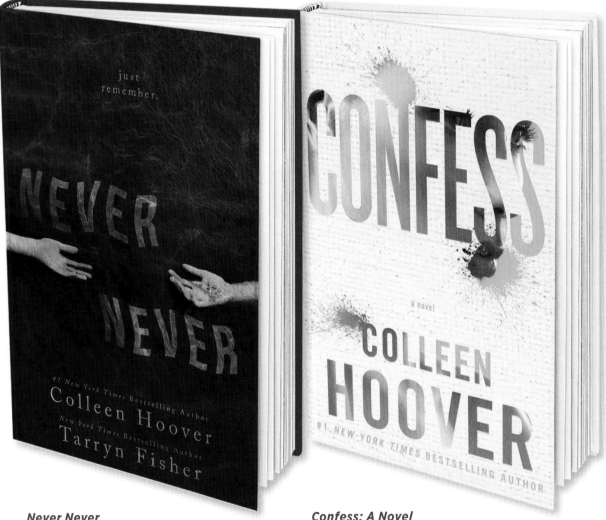

Never Never
by Colleen Hoover and Tarryn Fisher
January 21, 2015
She doesn't want to forget. He doesn't want to remember. Can they both get what they desire?

Confess: A Novel
by Colleen Hoover
March 10, 2015
To save his relationship, Owen must reveal his darkest secret. But what if the confession is worse than the sin?

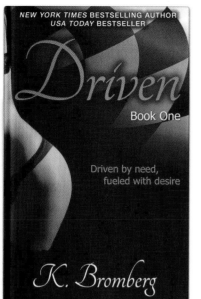

Driven
by K. Bromberg
Neither is the other's type, but Rylee Thomas and Colton Donavan may have just met each other's match.

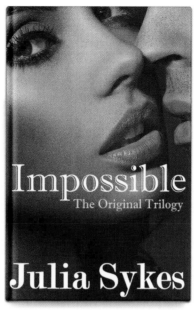

Impossible: The Original Trilogy
by Julia Sykes
After she's abducted, Claudia is torn between fear for her life and the feelings she's developing for her captor.

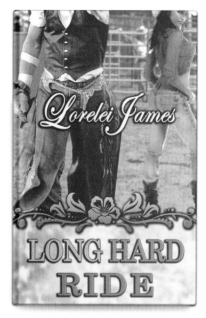

Long Hard Ride
by Lorelei James
One up-for-anything woman. Three hardworking, hard-living cowboys. One long, sexy summer break.

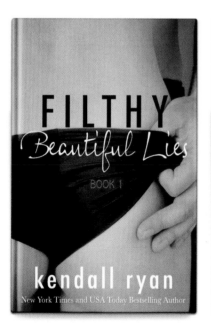

Filthy Beautiful Lies
by Kendall Ryan
Forced to auction off her virginity, Sophie Evans expects to be bought by a man with twisted desires. Enter: Colton Drake.

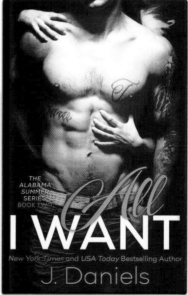

All I Want
by J. Daniels
Sexual tension and passions run rampant in this story of two people who are just too stubborn to say, "I need you."

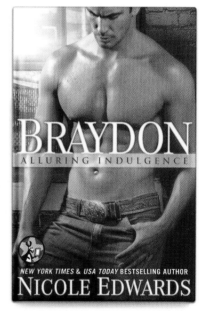

Braydon
by Nicole Edwards
Identical twins Braydon and Brendon share everything—even women—until Braydon meets Jessie, and his entire world shifts.

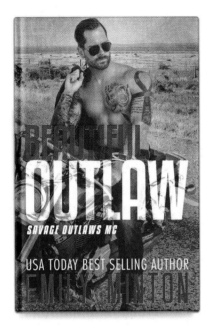

Beautiful Outlaw
by Emily Minton
After faking her death to escape an abusive husband, Laura must learn how to be herself again—with the help of biker Bowie.

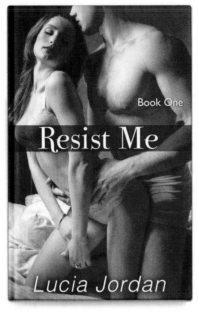

Resist Me
by Lucia Jordan
After snubbing him in college, Cheyanne reencounters Brett as her new boss. Will she take the chance to make up for her mistake?

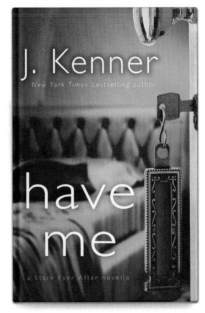

Have Me: A Stark Ever After Novella by J. Kenner
Damien and Nikki embark on their honeymoon. But their happily ever after is threatened when forces from their pasts return to haunt them.

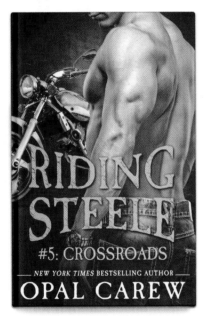

Riding Steele #5: Crossroads
by Opal Carew
Kidnapped by bikers, Laurie finds herself at the mercy of their powerful, sexy leader, Steele.

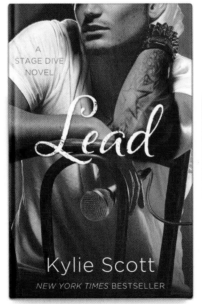

Lead: A Stage Dive Novel
by Kylie Scott
When Lena is hired to keep rocker Jimmy in line, his demanding nature might cause him to lose his saving grace.

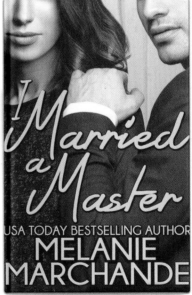

I Married a Master
by Melanie Marchande
Jenna must marry her kinky billionaire boss to secure his company and her job. But there's a catch: She must submit to him in every way.

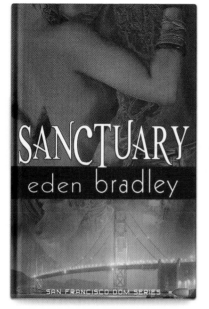

Sanctuary
by Eden Bradley
One night at a BDSM club was all it took for Devin to fall victim to its dark, erotic world and the enigmatic Shayne Vincent.

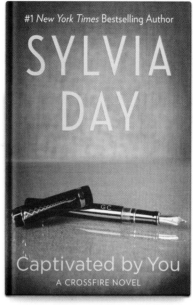

Captivated By You
by Sylvia Day
Facing dark pasts, Gideon and Eva must fight to save their marriage before their demons tear them apart forever.

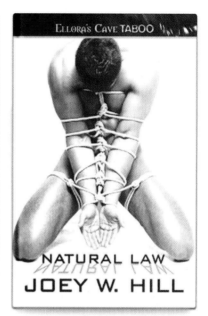

Natural Law
by Joey W. Hill
When Mac Nighthorse goes undercover as a male sub to find a murderess dom, he ends up finding more than just a lead in the case.

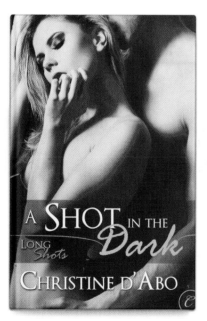

A Shot in the Dark
by Christine d'Abo
Paige can't resist the dominating yet selfless Carter. But will her history of abuse get in the way of unleashing her inner submissive?

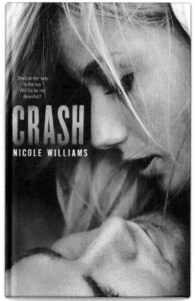

Crash
by Nicole Williams
Lucy Larson falls face first into the life of bad boy Jude Ryder. Every instinct tells her to run, but nothing will keep them apart.

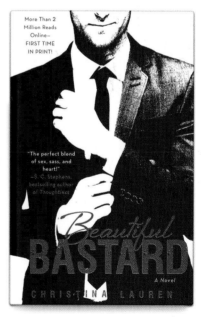

Beautiful Bastard
by Christina Lauren
A tenacious intern and rude boss act on a fiery attraction. But they must decide what they're willing to lose in order to gain each other.

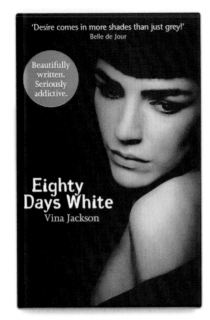

'Desire comes in more shades than just grey!'
Belle de Jour

Beautifully written. Seriously addictive.

Eighty Days White
Vina Jackson

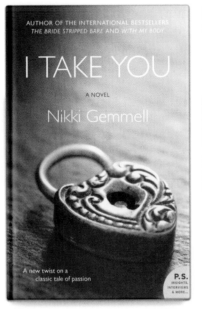

AUTHOR OF THE INTERNATIONAL BESTSELLERS
THE BRIDE STRIPPED BARE AND *WITH MY BODY*

I TAKE YOU

A NOVEL

Nikki Gemmell

A new twist on a classic tale of passion

P.S.
INSIGHTS,
INTERVIEWS
& MORE...

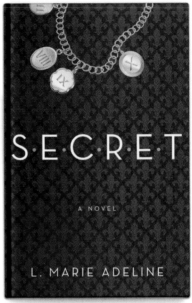

S·E·C·R·E·T

A NOVEL

L. MARIE ADELINE

Eighty Days White
by Vina Jackson
Lily meets Leonard and is whipped into a carefree world of passion and adventure. But will she accept the real woman she finds within herself?

I Take You
by Nikki Gemmell
After her husband, Cliff, gets into a ski accident, Connie's true nature is revealed when she must serve his every need.

S.E.C.R.E.T.
by L. Marie Adeline
Cassie's desires are brought to life when introduced to S.E.C.R.E.T., an underground club that turns women's fantasies into realities.

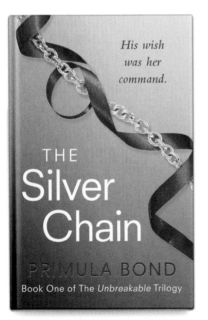

His wish was her command.

THE Silver Chain

PRIMULA BOND

Book One of The *Unbreakable* Trilogy

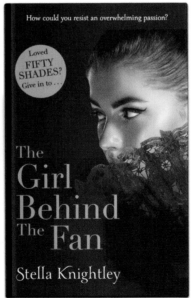

How could you resist an overwhelming passion?

Loved FIFTY SHADES? Give in to . . .

The **Girl Behind** The **Fan**

Stella Knightley

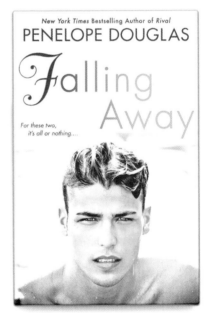

New York Times Bestselling Author of *Rival*

PENELOPE DOUGLAS

Falling Away

For these two, it's all or nothing....

The Silver Chain
by Primula Bond
Serena is symbolically bound to Gustav through a silver chain bracelet he gives her. But the tighter his hold grows, the closer his past comes to tearing them apart.

The Girl Behind the Fan
by Stella Knightley
Hurt and betrayed after her love affair with millionaire Marco ends, Sarah returns to an ex-boyfriend. But her love for Marco will not subside.

Falling Away
by Penelope Douglas
January 6, 2015
Avoiding him since high school, K.C. is now stuck in close quarters with the worst kind of temptation: Jaxon Trent.

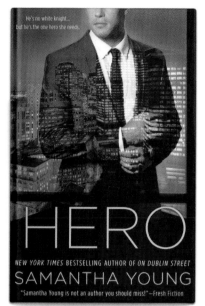

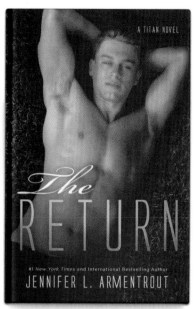

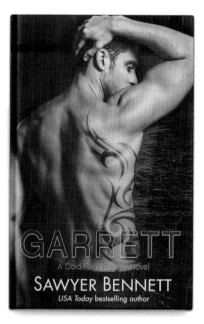

Hero
by Samantha Young
February 3, 2015
At odds with her father's dark secrets, Alexa meets Caine, and attempts to push her away bring them closer.

The Return
by Jennifer L. Armentrout
February 17, 2015
With a penchant for violence, Seth is now faced with a new challenge: restraint.

Garrett: A Cold Fury Hockey Novel
by Sawyer Bennett
February 17, 2015
A guy who lives for the next thrill. A girl who's not sure if she'll live through the next day.

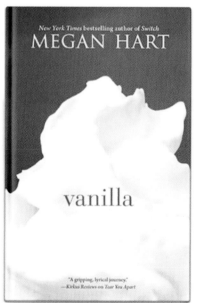

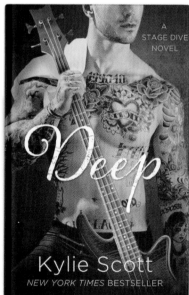

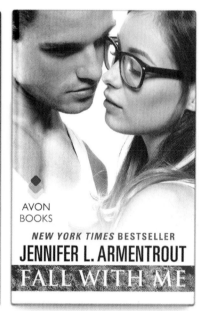

Vanilla
by Megan Hart
February 24, 2015
She always gets what she wants, but so does he. What happens when two lovers both want to be on top?

Deep: A Stage Dive Novel
by Kylie Scott
March 31, 2015
For Lizzy Rollins, what happens in Vegas doesn't always stay there.

Fall With Me
by Jennifer L. Armentrout
March 31, 2015
When a threat from the past returns, Roxy must rely on the man who's broken her heart more than once.

Fifty Trends of Grey
Jamie Dornan's Christian Grey hands over the keys of a brand new Audi to Dakota Johnson's Anastasia Steele. In July 2012, Audi reported an all-time record, a 28 percent sales increase from July 2011. Though it's not clear whether *Fifty Shades of Grey* was to blame (or thank), the spike in sales during that time also matched that of Brooks Brothers (for ties) and the bondage section in sex shops everywhere.

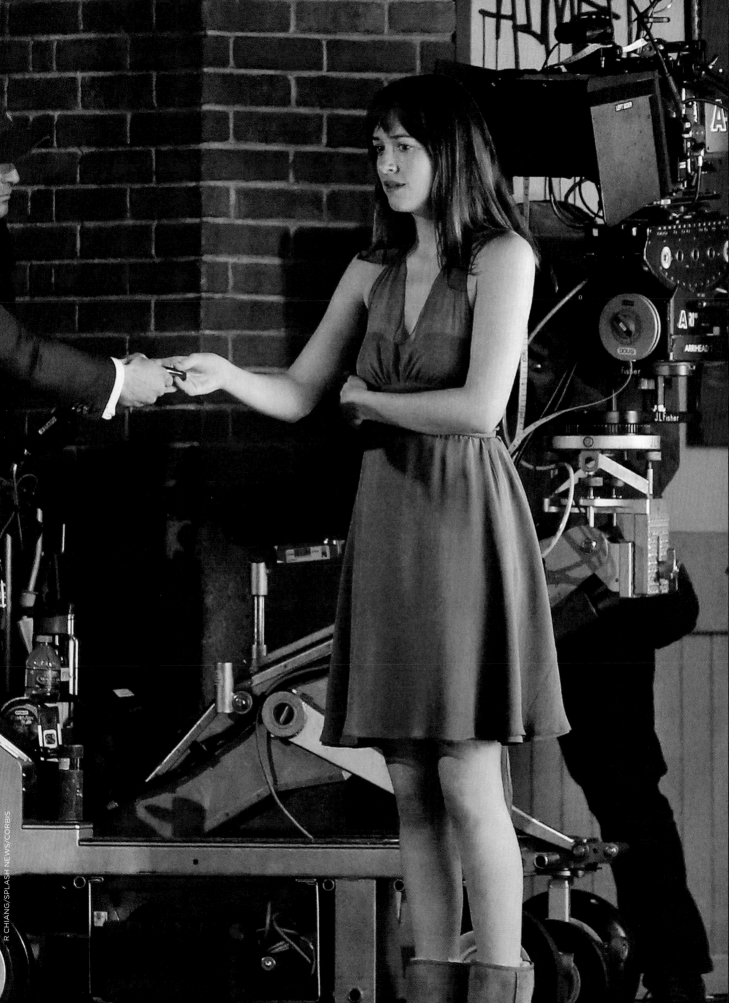

Stimulus Package
Sex toy sales skyrocketed from coast to coast in 2012 following *Fifty*'s break into the mainstream. San Francisco-based Good Vibrations saw its bondage sex toy sales increase 65 percent, and sales at New York-based adult toy store Babeland grew 40 percent.

THE
FIFTY
LIFE

EXPLORING BDSM

The story of one woman's journey to both sides of the paddle and back.

W hen I was 22, I took a job at a sex toy store owned by women. Naturally, I was sexually curious, and I quickly gained plenty of hands-on experience, both on the sales floor and in my personal life. I began to work my way through the shop's stock (we got an exceptional discount), starting with less intimidating plastic vibrators, then moving on to devices that looked space-aged and promised new experiences. But I never ventured as far as the "back wall," stacked with swaths of black leather, things with buckles and clasps and shiny metal implements. I learned from my co-workers that it was equipment used for something called BDSM, which stands for bondage, discipline

(or domination), sadism and masochism. I only knew this intellectually, having had no experience or—until this point—interest in what could be done with these types of toys. But having found satisfaction (both solo and with partners) in the devices I'd tried so far, I decided to get educated. First-hand.

I quickly discovered that I liked getting spanked. Harmless. Playful. Submissive. The impact of a light leather riding crop, stiff paddle or multi-tailed flogger on my bare behind would elicit bursts of joy. It started one night when a sweet but up-for-anything guy I was seeing gave my butt a few little swats. We weren't even having sex at the time, just goofing off. I was surprised—and pleased—by his initiative and excited by how good it felt. The innocent

Prop Master
Chloe still owns many of the implements she utilized during both her dom and sub phases, but she prefers to keep things less role-oriented.

"I QUICKLY DISCOVERED THAT I LIKED GETTING SPANKED. HARMLESS. PLAYFUL. SUBMISSIVE."

playing quickly turned steamy as he increased the intensity of his smacks, and I responded to each with a "thank you, sir." It seemed like the right thing to say.

Bondage was the natural progression. And I loved it—at first. With cuffs or rope and the use of a blindfold, my sensations were heightened. Normal, even boring sex changed with just a simple restraint. But this is where the excitement, the fun of doing something a little taboo, ended for me.

I didn't like the stinging pain of bamboo canes. Very flexible, the loud whoosh a cane makes as it cuts through the air precedes a concentrated A-bomb as it strikes the skin—even when used gently. I learned this the hard way when a lover wanted to roleplay as headmaster versus naughty schoolgirl and introduced me to the sensation of canes during the action. After lifting my plaid skirt and "assuming the position" (bent over with bottom in the air), I heard my punishment descend. For precisely one second I thought, "Hmm, that wasn't as bad as it sounded." Then the wave of pain settled in. I howled! Canes sneak up on you.

Gags further confirmed my limits. Soft, sexy material draped around my mouth was fine, but nothing could be less pleasing than a ball gag. The first time I was instructed to bite down on a big red rubber ball as it was fastened around my neck, I not only couldn't speak, I couldn't swallow. But I wanted to know my true limit. Soon, drool was dripping down my chest and I felt my tongue start to tingle. Not my idea of sexy. I made a "timeout" sign (our silent safe word or gesture) with my hands, and the gag was removed.

"Sorry." I apologized, embarrassed. "That made my tongue feel weird." I haven't used another gag since.

Being on the business end of a paddle, crop or blindfold was a great experience for me as a woman. A feminist. I wanted to see and feel this for myself. But, over time, I was drawn to the giving end of BDSM—weaving an elegant harness over a torso with rope, confidently strapping things on or commanding a submissive man to do what I wanted. It's not

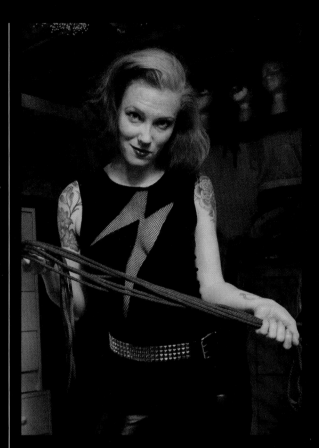

A Bevy of Subs The willing, submissive men Chloe encountered included one guy who wanted to eat her cigarette butts and another who was turned on by racial slurs regarding his Indian heritage.

something you learn in a book. It takes practice.

Armed with a sense of toughness I'd never felt before, at a friend's party I struck up a conversation with a cute, corporate-type guy my age. Talk turned to flirting, which led to chatting about how sexy this guy found powerful women. I took his number and after a couple of casual dates it came out that my new friend was into a certain kind of powerful woman—specifically, comic book she-villains. He had a particular fantasy about being kidnapped by Catwoman. Why not give it a try? I didn't have the ears, but I did have a latex catsuit. I really hammered it up, tossing a cape over his head and dragging him across the room, then tying him to a chair and giving him a

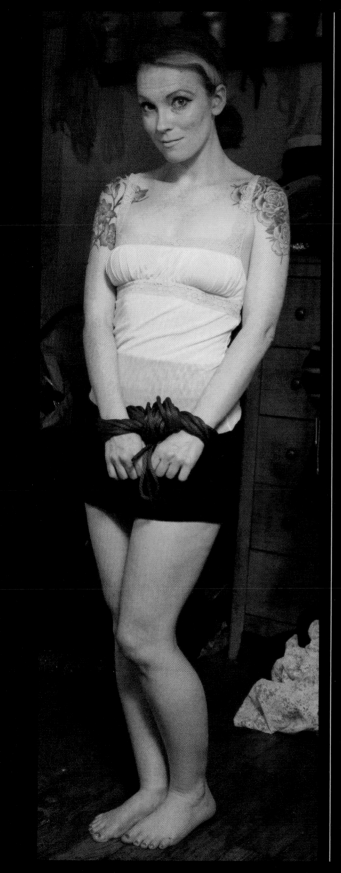

"I began to feel like what had started as a fun, sexy little adventure...had cracked open a Pandora's box of perversions."

thorough "interrogation" peppered with lots of purring. "You sound like a snake," he remarked, and I felt ridiculous. "Like Medusa! That's sexy," he continued, so I kept it up. I was happy with the experience, which was akin to an X-rated improv class. It was silly but exciting.

Others begged me to whiz on them; some got highly aroused being repeatedly told their above-average-sized member was actually tiny; some wanted to be kicked in the crotch. Hard. With my pointiest shoes on. I began to feel like what had started out a fun, sexy little adventure—my sexual liberation fantasy—had cracked open a Pandora's box of perversions I wasn't sure I could handle. Or wanted to. Tell a potential lover you've messed around with S&M and suddenly they're confessing their dream of being saddled up, groomed like a thoroughbred and presented in faux-dressage.

The truth is, I missed making out. And cuddling. Nobody who wanted to be spanked was after either. I was due for a break. Maybe I was "vanilla" after all. I'll occasionally entertain spanking (getting and giving) or a bout of naughty schoolgirl role play, and I don't regret my dip into the darker parts of the sexual psyche. I'm fascinated by the wildness of our collective sexual imaginations, and I support the desire to (safely, sanely and consensually) act on them. But I won't be participating.

STRUGGLE OF A SECRET SUB

Julie, a 31-year-old doctor, feels it's more important to keep her sexual tastes a secret than it is to find a real-life Christian Grey.

Why is it so important for you to keep your sexual preference hidden when it's obvious that it is more and more normalized?
Any sex anyone engages in is very private and may not be consistent with their public and professional roles. You might be a high-ranking executive and go home and have sex in front of your window. That's normal-ish, but it's still not consistent with your role as a leader and as an executive. Maybe it's absurd, but sex in and of itself, although everyone does it, is something deviant and private. You don't talk about it. It's not so dramatic to me—everyone is doing something a little deviant anyway—but I am extraordinarily paranoid about sexuality interfering with my career and my future success. I work in a clinical capacity, taking care of patients. Doctor stuff.

Have you noticed since the phenomenal success of *Fifty Shades* that your sexual proclivities are quickly becoming less taboo?
It does make it more acceptable in ways. When people hear more about [BDSM play] in a way that's digestible to them, it helps advance understanding of this type of sexuality. And maybe even an awareness of their own selves.

The D/s Dilemma
Sixty-one percent of women surveyed said they would classify themselves as more submissive, the remaining 39 percent sided with doms.

Do you think most women have a naughty side to them, even if only casually?

Most women I talk to are interested in being submissive to some degree. They want it, but not all the time. I've found that a woman wanting to be safely roughed up a little bit is pretty common. But that's also what's difficult for me because it's easy to find that, but it's not exactly what I want.

"I don't have time to be locked in a cage for 24 hours or kneel in a corner all night."

What is it you want?

Ideally, I'd want to marry someone who shared my sexual interests, as most people would. What happens to some people is the perfect person they find doesn't share their sexual interests but tolerates them. That won't work for me in a relationship. I'd need to be the sub to a master. But, ideally, he would also respect me. I know that sounds unusual. It's a monogamous, trusting relationship. He's just someone who I answer to. We both have similar career goals. A few years ago, I was engaged. I lived with someone for several years, and the plan was to get married. Probably because I'm in a conservative profession, it seemed like the natural next step. There were some fundamental incompatibilities, though, so we eventually broke off the engagement. It got to a point where I had so much control over this guy that I couldn't see him as a dominant man. Actually, I was kind of bossy in that relationship. Since then, I've come to realize that I can't be with so-called "vanillas." I need someone who is a little bit more feisty.

How does that play out during the day when you're caring for patients and being bossed around at home? Where does it end?

If a guy told me to clean the toilet, that's not really something that appeals to me. It's always going to be in the context of some kind of sexual game. I don't have time to be locked in a cage for 24 hours or kneel in a corner all night. But I was surprised to find in recent years that I like to extend it to some degree outside of the bedroom. Like at a restaurant, giving a scolding look if I do something wrong. Or, if we're walking across the street, instead of holding hands he is holding my wrist tightly, leading me across the street. Something like that is more subtle, not so extreme. Do I want someone to tell me what to do every single second of the day? No. I'm a junior doctor, so in the world of medicine, I'm kind of the bitch of the hospital. I don't feel like I have power as a doctor. I have a lot of responsibility, but I'd never feel like I'm the top of the chain. I don't have this image of being in a dominant role. But, even if I did, I think it's about stress relief. Regardless of what you do or what position you have, sex is always a good escape, in any person's life.

What would be an unusual request to a "normal" person but just fine with you?

Being used as a human coffee table.

Like wiping you with Pledge? Or more like setting a beer on your back?

Putting his feet up on my back. While nude. Staying still. That, to some people, sounds abnormal. It can be a very emotional, intense relationship to me. I could fall in love with a vanilla type of man, but it would be in a much less intense way. The mind needs to extend beyond the physical and the sexual.

What won't you do?

There are certain positions that have never been appealing to me. For instance, I'd never be on top. I mean I will do it, because I'm a submissive, but the man would have to be psychologically controlling me from the bottom, carefully instructing me. I want to be totally controlled. That's something subtle, but important. This requires a persona, a way of thinking. I cannot be in a relationship with someone who doesn't have that.

When was your first experience with this?

I was 19. I selected the guy I ended up losing my virginity to because when we were kissing, he shoved me up against a wall and started aggressively tonguing me. That's all it took. It was a very gradual awareness and realization.

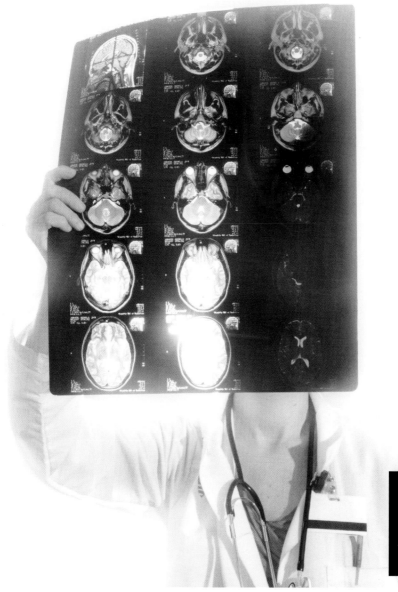

Head Examiner
Julie is aware enough of her own thought processes to know after just a few short questions whether or not she'll be sexually compatible with a partner.

When I started formally telling men about it, I found they're all into it on some level. If I would mention I like dominant men, then usually the guy would proceed accordingly with something benign, hair pulling, things that might not have been done initially. I was with a guy and said, "You've got to be a bit more rough, you've got to rough me up," and he said, "Well, I don't want to hurt you." I said, "But that's what turns me on. I like it." From then on he viewed me as if I must have been beaten as a child, which was silly. I realized he didn't think the way I need a partner to think. I'm a little bit beyond normal, but I'm not so extreme as to be considered a weirdo.

So is it really that hard to find a "Christian" or even a safe partner?

I find it very frustrating. I've tried to allude to it. Sometimes if I meet someone I ask, "What does D/s mean?" Some people who are not interested might know, but then I can kind of probe further. This is the problem, with most men, when they hear this, they are instantly interested. But I'm not interested in a fraud. They say it's something they're interested in, but it's not. Those guys are a dime a dozen. I want someone who needs it, who I can develop a relationship with. I don't want to offend people, I don't want to insult people. I just don't want to be judged, and I want to be able to find sexual partners without having to peruse shady online personals.

ANASTASIA'S SURVIVAL KIT

What started as drinks with friends just might end in unexpected bliss. Don't get caught without these items in your bag!

DIOR ADDICT GLOSS
Puffy, plump and always at the ready.
$31 *dior.com*

IPOD SHUFFLE
Add Kings of Leon and Snow Patrol to get a true musical taste of life with Christian and Ana.
$49 *apple.com/ipod-shuffle*

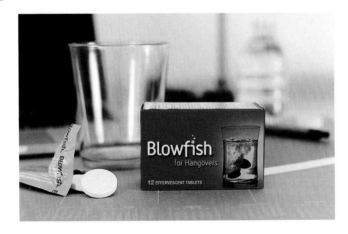

MIRACLE CURE **The best hangover remedy?**
Waking up swaddled in 1000 thread-count sheets and feather pillows at the Heathman Hotel followed by pancakes, eggs and bacon. Second best solution? Blowfish for Hangovers! Almost as good looking, just as reliable and even more soothing than Mr. Grey. Drop the tablets in water, drink when they've stopped fizzing and you'll be ready to face the day. Just $2 per hangover at CVS, Walgreens and *forhangovers.com*

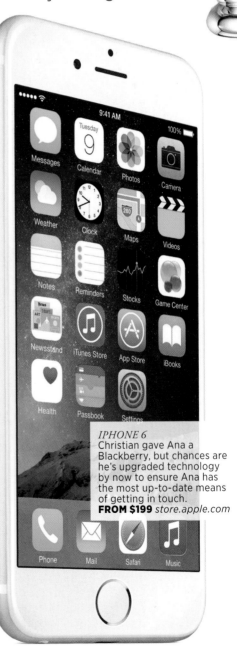

IPHONE 6
Christian gave Ana a Blackberry, but chances are he's upgraded technology by now to ensure Ana has the most up-to-date means of getting in touch.
FROM $199 *store.apple.com*

LE FUMEUR PANTY
Go from sensible to
sexy in a snap. See
below!
$20 *bexnyc.com*

*MINERALIZE CHARGED
FACE AND BODY LOTION*
This supple little number from
MAC is a great introduction to
crossing lines.
$33 *maccosmetics.com*

MIA 2
A portable aid for
when you want the job
done right. Its lipstick
shape allows for an
easy way to hide it in
plain sight.
$69 *lelo.com*

HANDCUFF KEYS
You never know when
you're going to need a
spare set.
$2 *handcuffwarehouse.com*

BLACK ELASTICS
Always keep an extra hair tie in
your purse just in case yours gets
snapped apart in the wild tussle
of erotic romance. You'll need it
to tame that morning-after hair.
$2.50 *remingtonproducts.com*

NEVER GET CAUGHT OFF-GUARD AGAIN!

STEP 1
Enjoy drinks with lady
friends.

STEP 2
Scope out worthy man-friends
who might pony up for Step 3.

STEP 3
Smile when man tells you he
owns a helicopter. Tell him
you'll just be a sec.

STEP 4
Realize you aren't
fully prepared for unexpected
awesome time.

STEP 5
Remedy "Monday undies"
with the BexNYC emergency
intimates switcheroo.

STEP 6
Walk side by side with the
confidence only this quick fix
can bring.

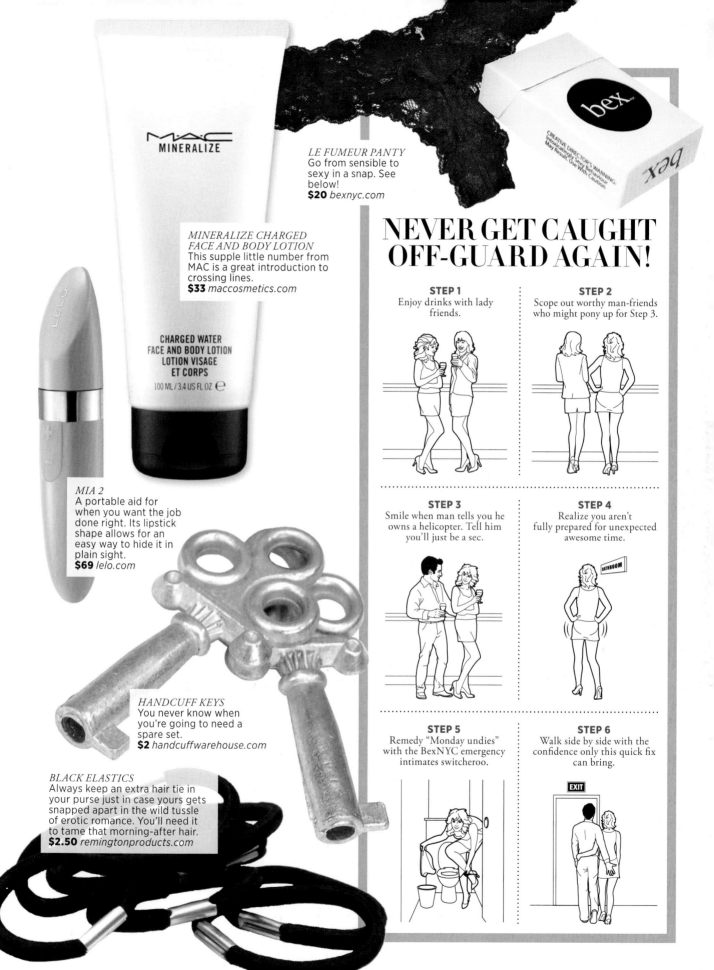

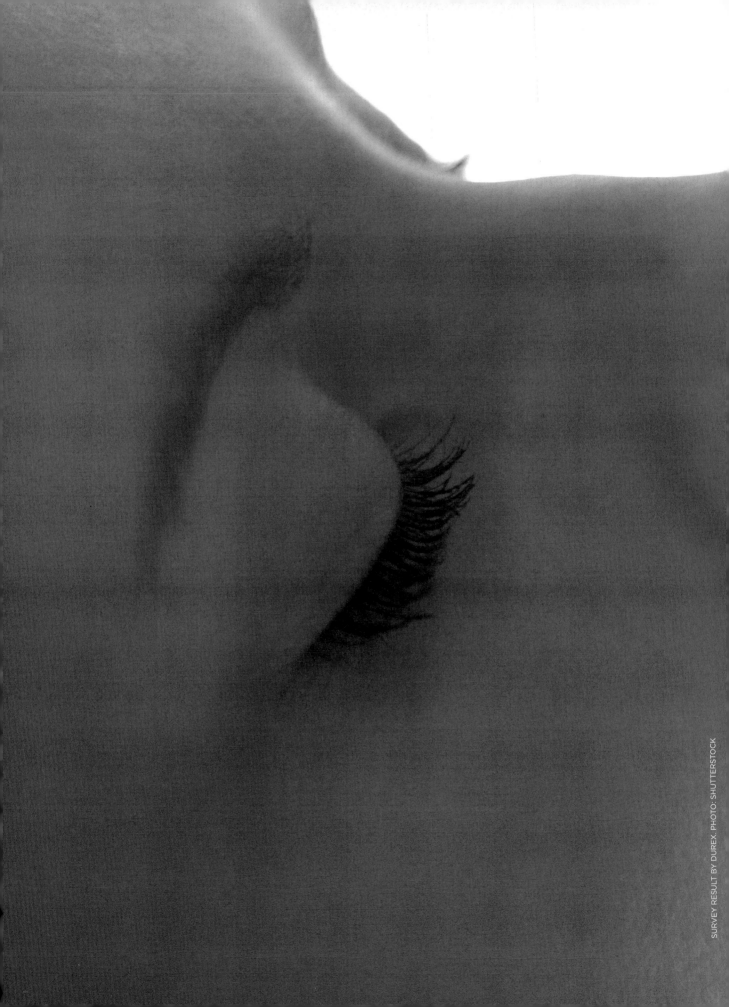

95% of women agree that getting closer means they can go further in fulfilling sexual fantasies.

TOY CLOSET

Must-have products that every lady should keep in her bag in case the night takes an unexpected turn.

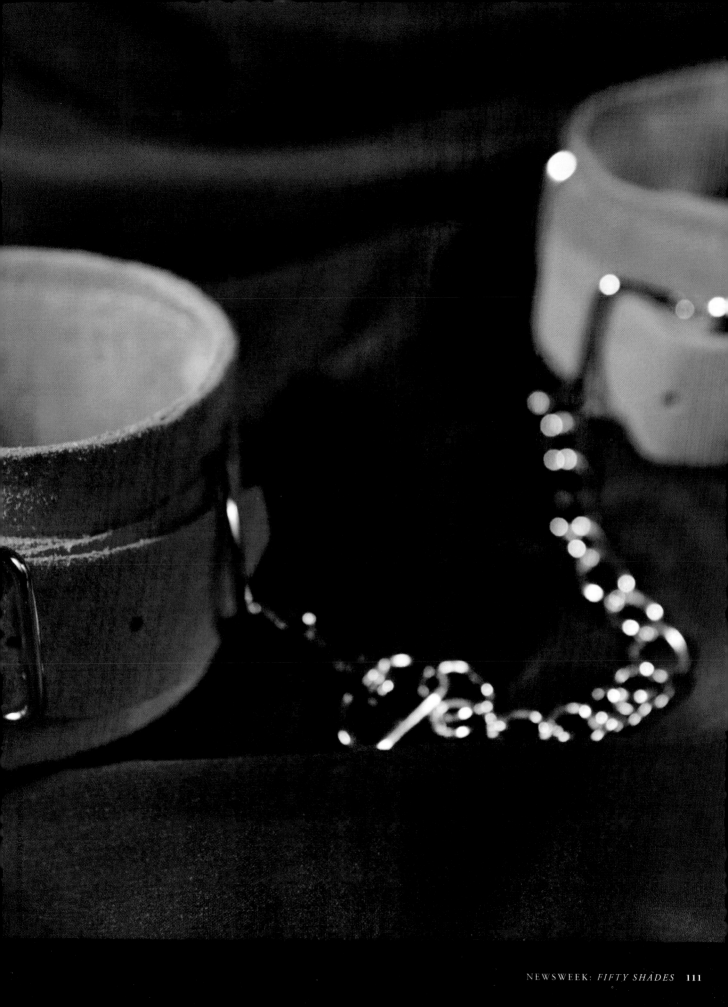

SUTRA CHAINLINK CUFFS
"Whenever things are getting a little boring in the bedroom, I take out these cuffs from their hiding place. No matter which one of us is bound, we both have a great time."
—Mary, 28 // Basking Ridge, NJ
$89 *lelo.com*

AMI PELVIC WEIGHTS
"I was nervous about them at first, but now I like to sneak them in before going to a movie theater or for a long car ride."
—Carrie, 24 // Chicago, IL
$70 *jejoue.com*

OLA VIBRATOR
"The Ola always responds to my touch and, unlike my boyfriend, gives me exactly what I want."
—Stephanie, 25 // Baton Rouge, LA
$149 *minnalife.com*

WE-VIBE II PLUS VIBRATOR
"Let's just say I'm glad it's rechargeable."
—Amanda, 34 // Tallahassee, FL
$218 *we-vibe.com*

BETTER THAN CHOCOLATE VIBRATOR
"It changes pulses based on the song that's playing, so it's like being teased by a drummer. I have a thing for drummers."
—Pamela, 21 // Portland, OR
$99 *shop.ohmibod.com*

ICICLES NO. 12
"I love how discreet this thing is. I accidentally left it out when my parents were over, and they complimented my 'beautiful sculpture.'"
—Jessica, 38 // San Francisco, CA
$80 *amazon.com*

SENSUA SUEDE WHIP
"This whip was a nice way for my boyfriend and me to ease into BDSM and explore our kinkier sides, and there are definitely no regrets!"
—Sandra, 22 // Buffalo, NY
$44 *lelo.com*

FORM 4 VIBRATOR
"Since I bought this, I don't mind so much when my man travels for business."
—Cheryl, 32 // Atlanta, GA
$145 *jimmyjane.com*

RABBIT HABIT ORIGINAL DELUXE VIBRATOR
"It's more than a toy. It's a relationship saver!"
—Kristin, 23 // Sandusky, OH
$92 *goodvibes.com*

TANGO VIBRATOR
"There are a lot of toys that are good for 'us time.' But this one's my go-to for 'me time.'"
—Melissa, 33 // New York, NY
$79 *we-vibe.com*

SEXY SHOP 101

Samantha Bard, co-owner of Shag, an erotic boutique in Brooklyn, offers up a few tips to the first-time sex toy shopper.

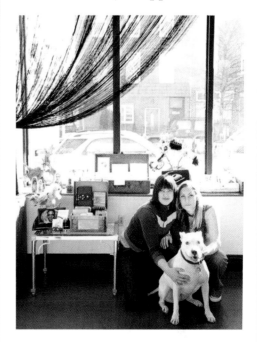

BE COMFORTABLE
Choose a place you feel comfortable going into. At Shag, we have a whole wall of windows that allow you to see out—and allow you to see in—which may sound daunting if you think about a sex shop. But we don't even consider ourselves a sex shop. We're a sexy shop.

GO SMALL
Smaller boutiques test all of their products and we are knowledgeable about everything we sell, whereas the bigger stores might not be as well-versed in all of the products they sell. If you want to be really educated on what you're buying, it's a better idea to go to a smaller boutique.

GO AT YOUR OWN SPEED
The first question I ask is, "Do you own any toys?" And if you say yes, we take it from there. If you say no, then we talk about if you like external stimulation versus internal. Once you find out what you like, we can talk about things that can really push your sex life.

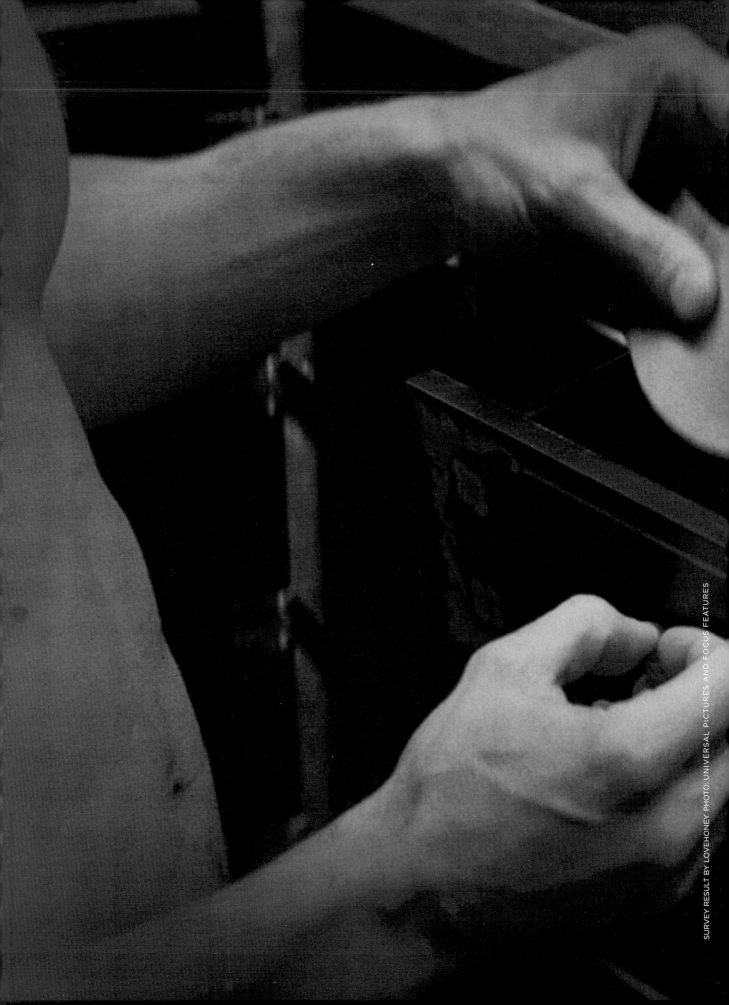

69% **of 2,500 people surveyed said they had** played with blindfolds.

TSA-APPROVED TOYS

The airport security squad's website is vague about which erotic items you're allowed to take on a plane, so one reporter decided to find out firsthand.

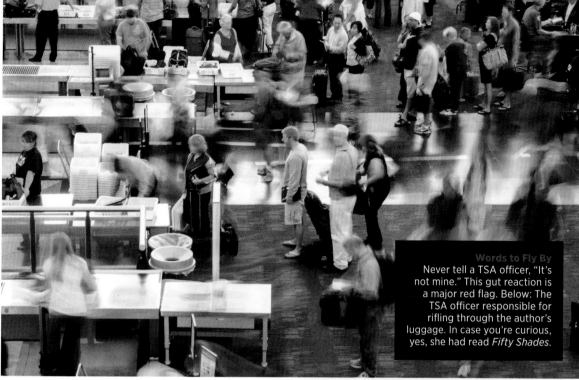

Words to Fly By
Never tell a TSA officer, "It's not mine." This gut reaction is a major red flag. Below: The TSA officer responsible for rifling through the author's luggage. In case you're curious, yes, she had read *Fifty Shades*.

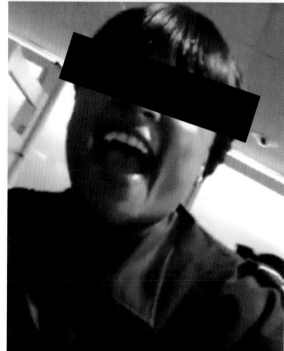

There are tons of things you can't or shouldn't take on a plane: Firearms. Snakes. Your teething infant. But the law is less clear when it comes to sex toys. Sure, it would be tough to cause an in-flight disruption with a riding crop, but you can imagine it. Handcuffs aren't necessarily a weapon, but they could theoretically be used in nefarious ways at 35,000 feet. I decided the only way to know which toys could be taken aboard an airplane would be to fill a suitcase full of them and take a flight.

I approached the security line at New York's LaGuardia airport with a smile on my face, a song in my heart and a bounty of pleasure aids in my carry-on. I'd packed my bag with the usual necessities for a one-night road trip, as well as a few items you might only pack if you were going to a *Fifty Shades* convention. I breezed through the metal detector with the confidence of a man who never wears a belt and has no piercings or pins in his bones. I waited dutifully for my baggage to pop out the other side of the X-ray machine, but started to sweat (as we all do) when my suitcase was flagged by a TSA employee.

"Bag check…" she announced as she brought my bag of tricks over toward the end of the conveyor line. "Is this yours, sir?"

"Yes," I looked at the floor. My inner goddess was equally nervous. "Do you have handcuffs in your bag?" she asked quietly. I couldn't tell if she was trying to protect my identity as a Federal Marshal or keep the conversation we were about to have about my kinky sex-fiendery between the two of us.

"Do you have handcuffs in your bag?" she asked.

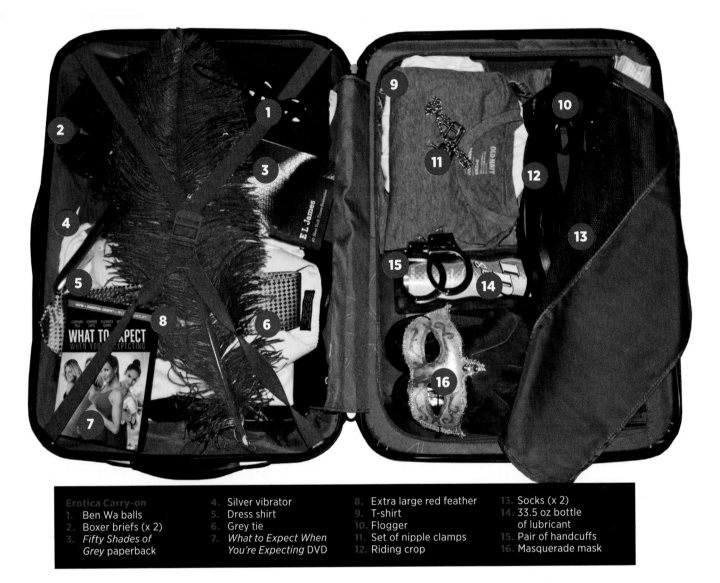

Erotica Carry-on
1. Ben Wa balls
2. Boxer briefs (x 2)
3. *Fifty Shades of Grey* paperback
4. Silver vibrator
5. Dress shirt
6. Grey tie
7. *What to Expect When You're Expecting* DVD
8. Extra large red feather
9. T-shirt
10. Flogger
11. Set of nipple clamps
12. Riding crop
13. Socks (x 2)
14. 33.5 oz bottle of lubricant
15. Pair of handcuffs
16. Masquerade mask

"I do," I said without much gravitas. Her eyes blinked. I'm not sure what her thoughts were, but her face passed a simple judgment. "Sex fiend it is," I thought.

She deftly removed the red, two-foot-long feather from my bag and gingerly placed it on the conveyor belt. "Gotta be careful with that," she smiled.

"Yeah," I nodded, subconsciously pleading the Fifth and saying as little as possible. If she'd asked a direct question such as, "What's this for?" or, "Why do you want to take this on a plane?" or, "What's your safe word?" I might have responded differently. But because she was invading my bag as opposed to my personal privacy, she mercifully kept the questions to a minimum.

At this point a few other TSA officers were craning their necks to see what else I had in my bag. The agent delicately maneuvered around my paperback copy of *Fifty Shades of Grey* and knowingly nodded, a smile on her face. It was at once clear to me that she had read the book and that she thought she might be part of some would-be viral event. Then she put her hands on the one item that had brought us to this impasse in the first place: a 33.5 ounce, economy-sized bottle of lube.

"You can't take this on the plane" she said matter-of-factly.

Before saying something stupid like, "But that's not mine," which would surely have escalated the whole affair to heavy pat-down proportions, I caught myself and played the fool. "But it's wrapped. It's brand new. It has a plastic wrapper on it."

"You still can't take it," she scolded, crossing her arms. I wondered how many times a day she had this conversation.

She set it aside and did a quick visual check of everything else I had in my bag. "So all of this other stuff is OK?" I asked, indicating the flogger, the handcuffs and the unopened *What to Expect When You're Expecting* DVD.

"Yes, that's no problem," she said. "Do you want to check your bag?" she asked, giving me the impression that she was keenly aware of how expensive a giant bottle of lube is. I declined. I told her she could keep it, but she politely (and very professionally) explained that TSA policy prevented her from accepting.

There are plenty of questions you ask when packing for a flight knowing you'll soon face the judgemental eyes of the TSA. Can I take my razor? What's the policy on hair gel? How many condoms is too many condoms? But most of the items I thought would raise some eyebrows—the flogger, the handcuffs—weren't the reason my bag was searched. According to the TSA, the only dangerous item in my suitcase was the thing that is generally regarded to be the safest in the bedroom: the lubricant. I verified this fact by going through security at Minneapolis-St. Paul International airport with the same items in my carry-on, minus the Costco-sized bottle of go-grease. No one on the other side of the X-ray screen blinked. My bag wasn't searched. In some ways, I felt short-changed.

Which is to say, if you're planning a trip but are worried your bag will make you look like a traveling sex-toy salesperson, don't panic. Just make sure everything else in your bag is in total compliance. Be overly careful. Pack your liquids separately, and remove anything from your bag that might appear to be some kind of vessel. (This includes your vibrator shaped like a shampoo bottle.) TSA employees are just doing their job, and they will avoid an embarrassing situation more often than not. If nothing in your bag is dangerous, they'll leave you and your feather-fetish alone.

And, in a pinch, if your bag is selected for a random search, don't panic. Never say something like, "What handcuffs?" Just tell them you are, in fact, a traveling sex toy salesperson. Offer them a discount. Chances are they'll send you on your way faster than you can say, "How many nipple clamps do you need?"

HIDDEN TOYS

Don't want judgemental looks from TSA officials? Never fear! Your guide to TSA-proof sex toys is here.

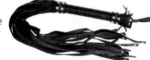

Lube
As long as the container is 3.4 ounces or less, you're all clear.

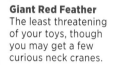

Flogger
Accepted, but to be safe, pack it in your checked luggage.

Giant Red Feather
The least threatening of your toys, though you may get a few curious neck cranes.

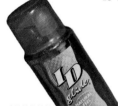

Riding Crop
Safe when traveling, but to avoid an awkward TSA encounter, don't pack it in your carry-on.

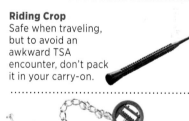

Nipple Clamps
NSFW, but definitely A-OK with the TSA.

Vibrators
Removing the batteries and limiting its length to 7 inches will ensure you don't get stopped.

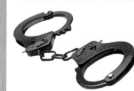

Handcuffs
Whether they're fuzzy, leather, have buckles or are bedazzled, handcuffs are approved.

91% **of men agree** *sex is better* **with someone who wants only you.**

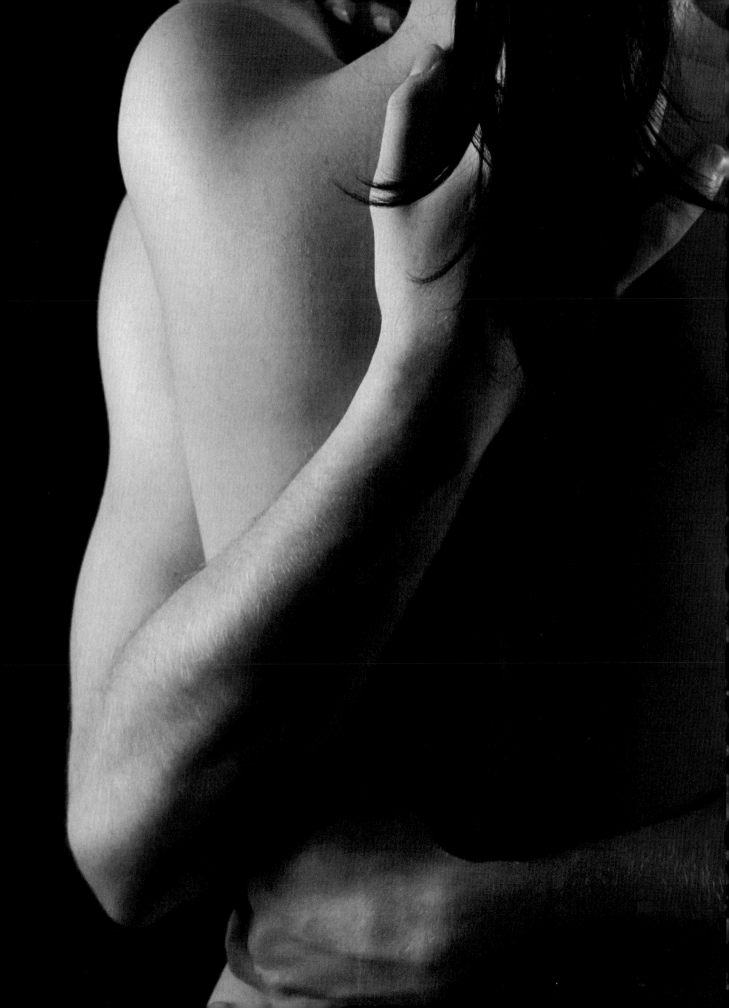

ROMANCE ENHANCED

We interviewed couples in different stages of their relationships to find out how the book has brought them closer and learned about candid bedroom fails, sex tricks revamped and an unexpected Greybie.

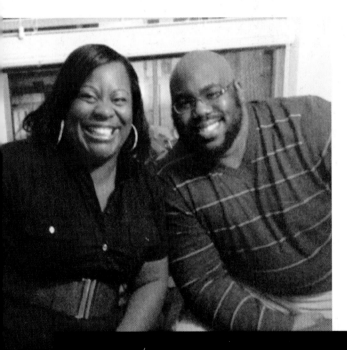

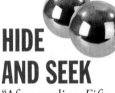

HIDE AND SEEK

"After reading *Fifty Shades of Grey*, I got really curious about those Ben Wa balls that Christian gives to Anastasia. So I tried them one time, all alone. Unfortunately, I lost them 'inside' and needed to take a trip to my gyno."—Deb

GIRLS JUST WANT TO HAVE FUN

"My wife and I met a married couple that we were attracted to. We'd go out to dinner, have a few drinks and then the men would watch the wives make out. It was a real turn-on…until our wives wouldn't let us join in."—Dan

LORI, 42 AND NATHANIEL, 33
Married // Pine Hill, New Jersey

Do you remind each other of the characters from the book?
Lori He might be more like Christian if I allowed him to use handcuffs.
Nathaniel I don't want her to be like Ana. Not many men want a woman they can completely control.

Has reading it improved your sex life?
Nathaniel We were already pretty active.

However, it did give us ideas for trying new things in the bedroom.
Lori We bought some his and hers KY Gel. We had a very active sex life, but [after reading *Fifty*] it was like, "Come on, get on top of me."

Had either of you considered some of the kinkier stuff in the book before reading it?
Nathaniel I am a true freak, so I'd thought of some of the stuff, but most women aren't willing.
Lori We did use the tie thing for my wrists.
Nathaniel She couldn't move and bumped her head on the headboard.

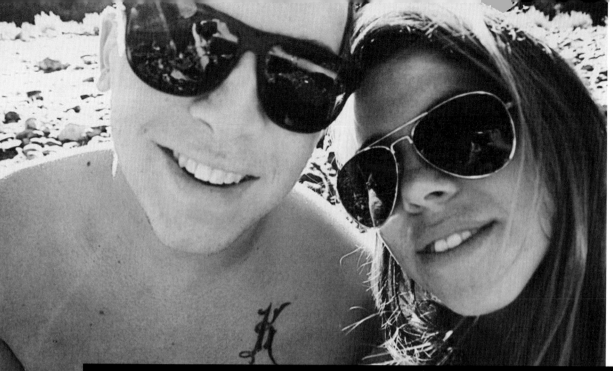

HAILEY, 22 AND MAX, 22
Dating // Arcata, California

What did you like about the book?
Hailey The storyline! It was scandalous and refreshing. At times, I skimmed over the sex scenes, especially in *Fifty Shades Darker* because it was suspenseful and more entertaining than reading how Anastasia's inner goddess was doing backflips again and again.

Has reading it changed your sex life?
Hailey This summer was the beginning of my long-distance relationship with Max, and it curbed some of the loneliness. My dreams became more sexually vivid and I caught myself fantasizing more. I saw him a few weeks ago, and I think having a more profound sexual imagination enhanced our sex life. I was also more excited since I'd only been reading about sex over the summer, and now I was finally getting some!

Did you try anything from the book?
Hailey We have. It was awesome. He was hesitant to continue and was shocked when I didn't stop him. It was like, "Whoa, where did that come from?"

VOLVO Y.O.L.O.

"My boyfriend and I had gone on a weekend trip with his family, but we finally had some alone time on the drive back. We were both pretty antsy since we hadn't been able to get frisky in a few days. Something about the barren scenery must have turned me on, so I went full 'bathtub scene' on him as we zipped along the highway. We soon deduced from the blue lights and sirens that were quick to follow us that not only was the road less deserted than we thought, but my oral skills had given him a lead foot, and we were going well over the speed limit. The poor guy had to stand on the side of the road and get a ticket in sneakers and a hand-towel while I laughed from the passenger seat."—Alex

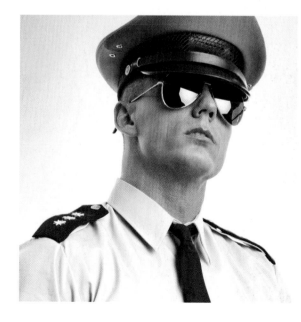

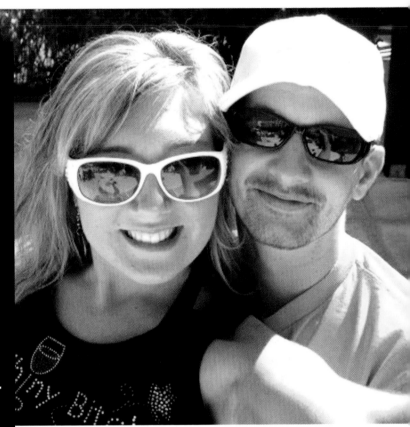

AMANDA, 25 AND ANDY, 30
Married // Minneapolis, Minnesota

Did you both read *Fifty Shades of Grey*?
Amanda He doesn't read, unless it's something online related to cars, news or hockey. E L James wasn't the first woman to write a racy romance novel, but I feel like she wrote the perfect book.

On a scale of 1–10, how would you describe the state of your sex life before you read the book?
Andy Before Amanda read them, I'd give it a 7.
Amanda A 7? We had enough to keep each other happy and satisfied, but there's always room for more!

Do you think reading it has improved your sex life?
Amanda A month after the release of *Fifty Shades Darker* we found out we were expecting. The book probably made getting in the mood easier!
Andy It's still a 7 for me.
Amanda We're working on getting it to 10.

Have you tried anything specific from the book?
Amanda I did purchase Ben Wa balls to try them out. Our 2-year-old found them in the "naughty drawer" in our bedroom and started to play with them thinking they were a toy. Not a proud moment.

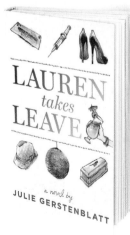

COMPILED BY JULIE GERSTENBLATT, WHO WRITES ABOUT THE DEMANDS OF MOTHERHOOD AND WIFEDOM IN MODERN SUBURBIA. HER FIRST NOVEL, LAUREN TAKES LEAVE, IS A TALE OF WOMEN ON THE VERGE, AVAILABLE THROUGH AMAZON.COM.

FIELDS OF YELLOW

"One time in college, my girlfriend and I decided to explore our adventurous side and have sex on the 50-yard-line of the football field. The Astroturf was wet when we laid down, but we didn't let that stop us. After we did the deed and put on our clothes, we realized from the smell that the moisture on the ground wasn't from sprinkler water. Apparently, peeing on the field is a fraternity ritual we weren't aware of."—Liam

SPANK YOU VERY MUCH

"A few years back, I was hooking up with this girl who really liked being spanked. So we were going at it and every time I spanked her she would say she wanted it harder. I complied and tried to give her a really hard one and tragically ended up catching one of my man-jewels between her cheek and my hand so hard that my knees gave out and I fell over. It wasn't the last time we hooked up, but it was probably one of the most memorable. I've since been working on my aim."—Rob

KITTY GLITTER

"While vacationing at my sister's house, I had a medical issue and went to see her gynecologist. When I saw an aerosol can of deodorant in her bathroom closet, I sprayed a little on my lady-space. When the doctor examined me, he said, 'Fancy.' I didn't know what he meant until I got changed for bed, realizing the spray I'd used all over my down-there-hair was actually Halloween hair glitter." —Wendy

HARD TO GET

"I tried to surprise my boyfriend by wearing real garters with stockings. He got so turned on when he saw me in them that he was like, 'I have to have you now.' But 'now' turned into quite a while later, because I'd mistakenly put the undies on under the garter belt."
—Joanne

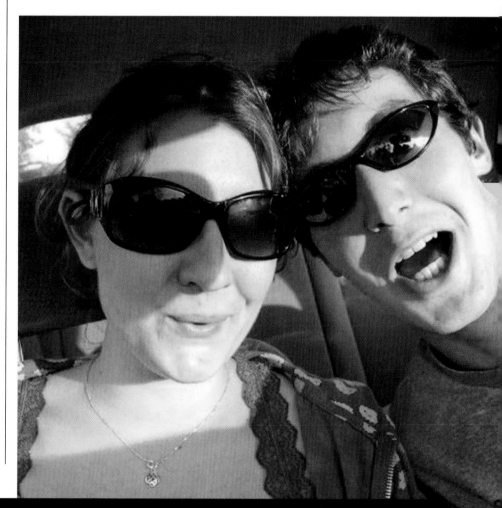

MICHELLE, 21 AND JOHN, 22
Dating // Philadelphia, Pennsylvania

Do you think reading *Fifty Shades* has improved your sex life?
Michelle Reading it made me more bold. I'm more inclined to open myself up more to sex.
John After Michelle read it, she seemed more interested in sex. More attentive. So I guess it works for girls.

Did the book inspire you to try anything new?
Michelle The only thing I had ever thought about was being tied up and tying my boy up.
John I am NOT going into detail about that.
Michelle Well, as it turns out, he gets panic attacks when he is tied up. He had some pretty nasty red marks on his wrists for quite awhile. And it was over the summer so he wasn't too thrilled about wearing long sleeves during the hot weather. Whoops!

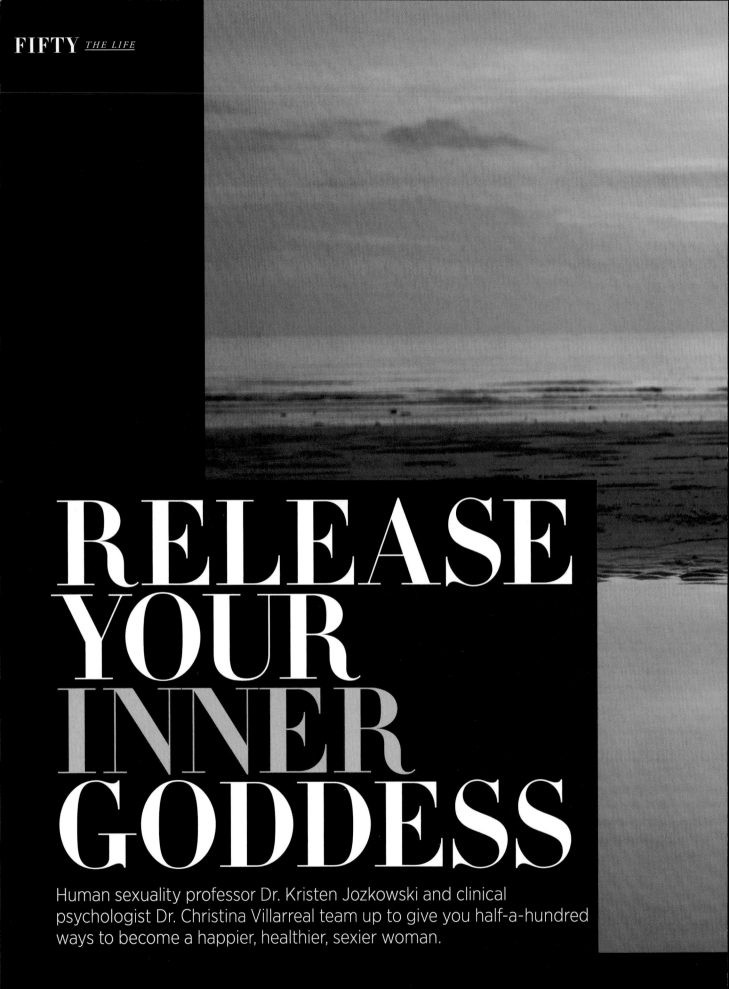

RELEASE YOUR INNER GODDESS

Human sexuality professor Dr. Kristen Jozkowski and clinical psychologist Dr. Christina Villarreal team up to give you half-a-hundred ways to become a happier, healthier, sexier woman.

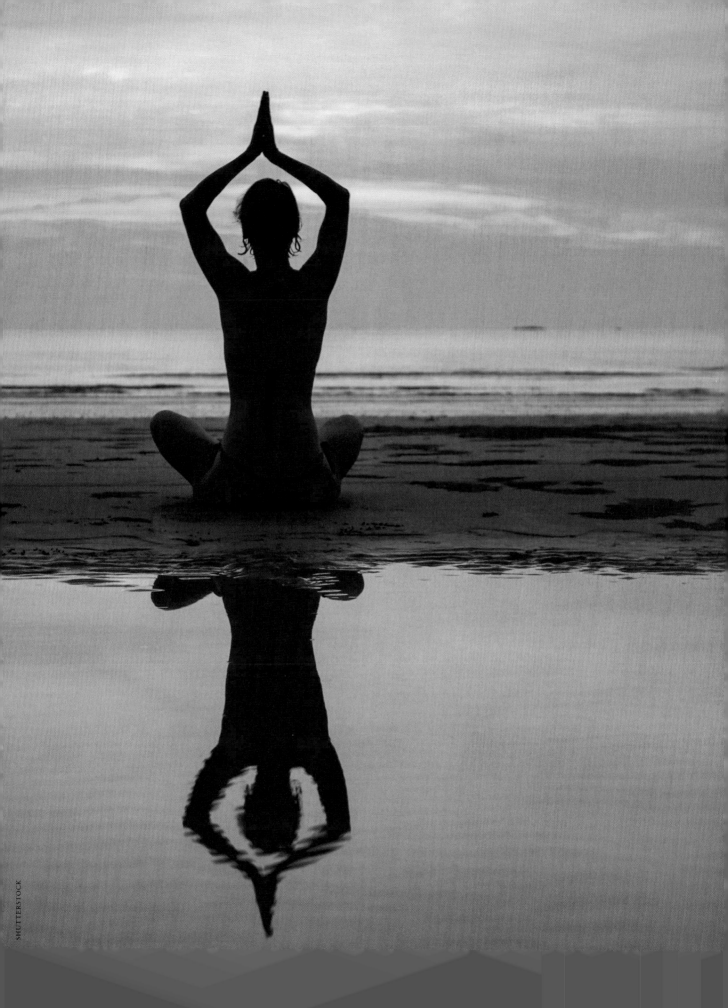

GET ACTIVE

"When women exercise they tend to feel better about themselves whether or not they've lost weight, gained weight, are big or small, have large breasts or small breasts. You can say, 'I feel good about my body because I'm doing healthy things for it.'" —Dr. Jozkowski

1 TAKE A YOGA CLASS
Yoga improves flexibility and posture and strengthens your muscles. Plus, it helps you slow down and tune in to your body, so you can bend and stretch your way to loving the way you look and feel.

2 GO FOR A RUN
Studies have shown running can reduce your chances of getting the common cold or even cancer. Additionally, adults who exercise on a regular basis are usually happier than those who don't. So crack a smile, throw on some sneaks and take a relaxing jog. Christian would approve.

3 TAKE A SPINNING CLASS
Want to be a lean, mean, biking machine? Spinners can burn 500 to 800 calories in only 45 minutes. This fad is equal parts dance party and communal therapy session, so you'll have a blast while blasting calories. It's also a great way to build up your stamina (also Christian-approved).

4 TAKE A HIKE
Research shows hiking in the countryside can reduce depression and boost self-esteem. So throw together some trail mix, grab a water bottle and take a breath of fresh air.

5 TRY A BELLY DANCING CLASS
Belly dancing is not only fun, but it's a great form of exercise. This healthy and exhilarating dance improves joint flexibility, circulation and reduces stress. It also impacts major muscle groups, including your legs, thighs, abs, upper arms and back.

6 POLE PARTY
Pole dancing classes may seem intimidating, but make it a group trip and treat your girlfriends. They're structured to build a strong mind and physique with a mix of cardio and strength training that unleashes your sexy side!

7 FLAUNT YOUR GREEN THUMB OUTDOORS
Did you know you can burn as many calories in 45 minutes gardening as you can with 30 minutes of aerobics? It's true. So get outside and get a little dirty.

8 STRAIGHTEN UP
Studies show individuals who maintain good posture throughout the day are often more confident and positive-minded than those who don't. Plus, good posture prevents unwanted back pain and requires that your abs stay fully engaged, toning without you even knowing it.

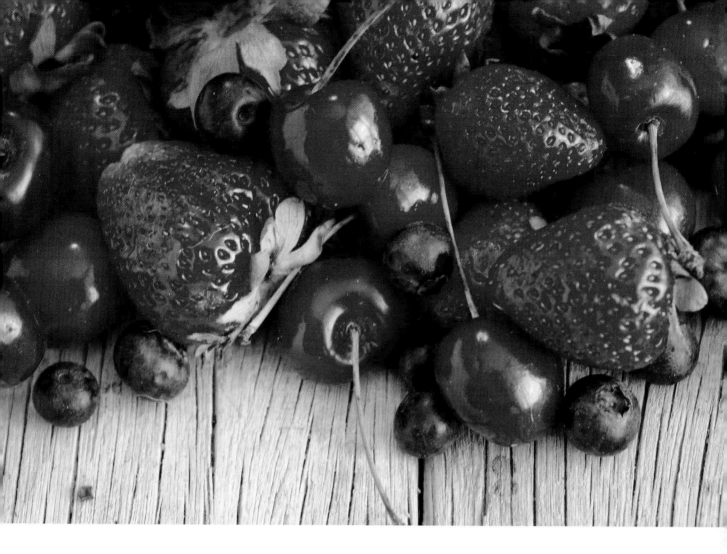

EAT RIGHT

Though you may not have Christian Grey to monitor your food intake, eating healthy is the simplest step toward feeling sexy.

9 BERRY SPECIAL SNACK

Fresh berries have been proven to infuse dull and dreary skin with brightness and color. Throw blueberries in your morning cereal, or toss some strawberries on a salad for a fruity kick.

10 GET NUTTY

Nuts contain fiber, good fats and protein—the perfect nutritional combo to awaken a youthful glow in your skin. Snack on walnuts, almonds and pumpkin seeds (a noted aphrodisiac!) to unleash soft, supple skin.

11 ADD A CHERRY ON TOP

These lush, red fruits are nutritional powerhouses, packed with antioxidants that aid in the prevention of cancer and heart disease. They're also rich in vitamins C and E, potassium and magnesium, iron, folate and fiber. Why not have two?

12 EAT AVOCADOS

Not only creamy and delicious, avocados are a huge source of fiber. Fiber helps prevent heart disease, high blood pressure and certain types of cancer.

13 MUNCH ON CHOCOLATE

Chocolate isn't always bad for you. In fact, studies show dark chocolate can help prevent heart disease, improve your mood and protect your skin. So indulge! Just make sure to limit yourself to no more than 3 ounces of the sweet stuff per day.

14 GO WILD WITH SALMON

Wild salmon, not farm-raised, is one of the top omega-3 fatty acid foods. It will keep your skin looking fresh and moisturized, plus the selenium it contains protects from sun exposure. For a tasty dinner, try a salmon burger or coat a salmon fillet in oil and herbs and throw it on the grill!

15 GET HOT WITH CHILES

Throw chiles inside a whole wheat veggie wrap for a tasty kick and a sexy spike. Chiles contain capsaicin, a chemical that increases blood flow and triggers the release of mood-enhancing endorphins that naturally amp your libido.

16 ROOT FOR MACA

Scientific studies show maca root can increase stamina, boost libido and combat fatigue. This plant contains p-methoxybenzyl isothiocyanate, the difficult-to-pronounce chemical responsible for its aphrodisiac effects. Toss maca root powder in a smoothie or a glass of water and drink up!

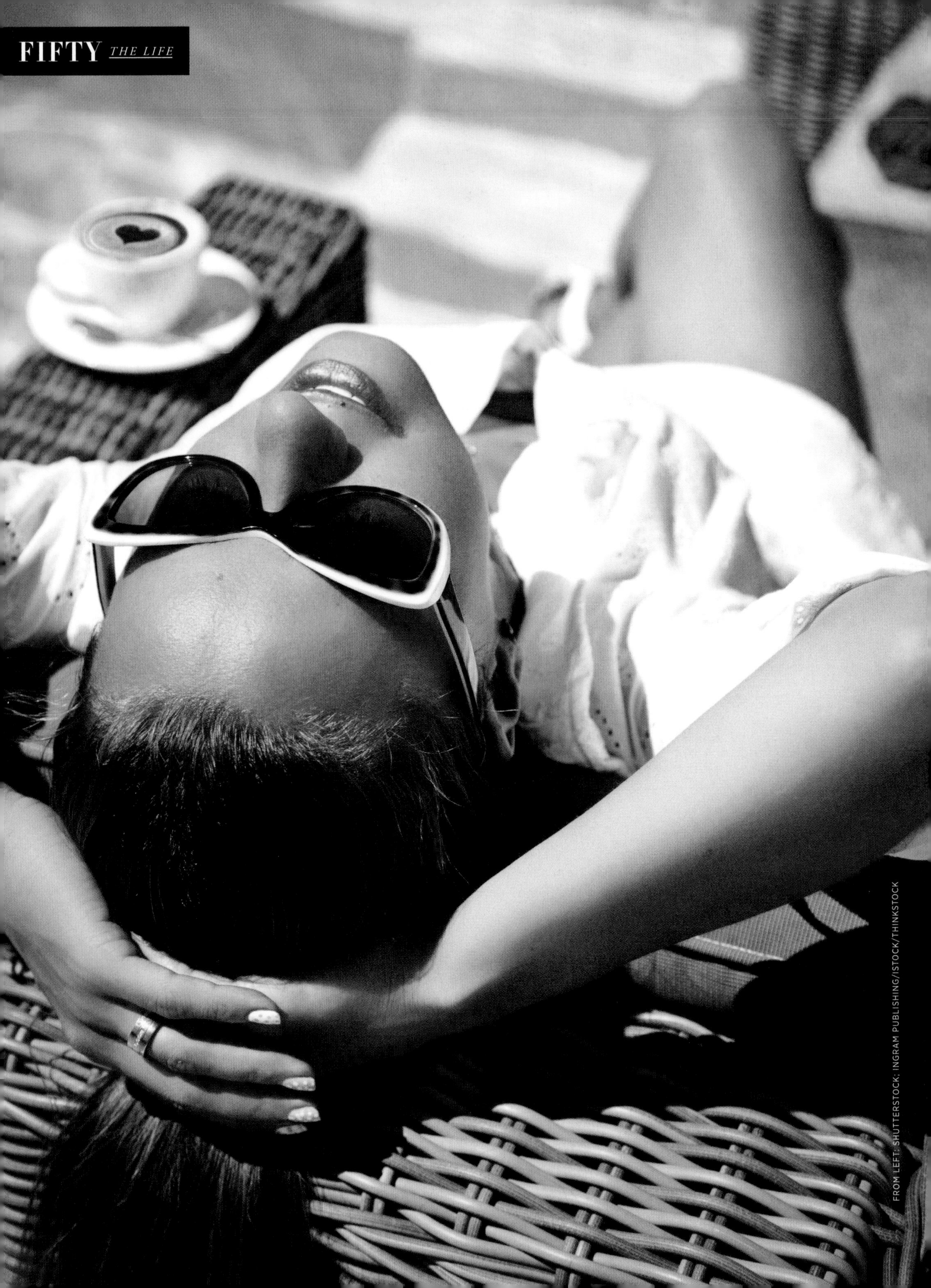

FROM LEFT: SHUTTERSTOCK; INGRAM PUBLISHING/ISTOCK/THINKSTOCK

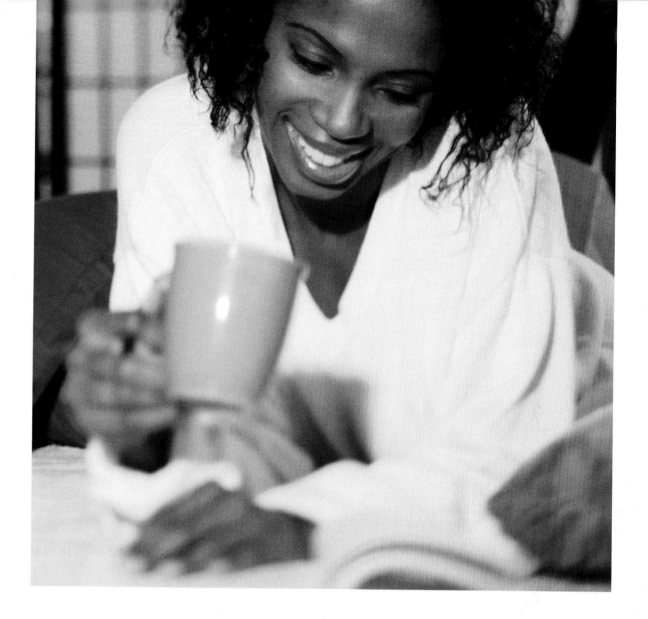

HAVE "ME TIME"

Before you can introduce your inner goddess to your man, you must first get to know her yourself.

17 GET COOKING
Home cooking can be an excellent stress reliever, plus it's a great way to manage exactly what you're putting into your body. Try whipping together a *Fifty Shades* staple, pasta alle vongole (see recipe on page 147), or just stick with Ana's favorite, pancakes and eggs.

18 REFLECT AND RELAX
Need a moment of peace? Take a bubble bath. Not only does it provide an excellent environment for relaxation, but the suds you choose can affect your mood. Add some lavender- or vanilla-scented bubbles to create tranquil energy, and use peppermint or citrus to feel energized.

19 HIT THE BOOKS
Just like muscles, the brain benefits from a good workout. Studies show the mental activity of reading keeps your memory sharp and your mind focused, especially as you age. (See page 88 for suggestions on new reads.)

20 SEEK SUNSHINE
When our bodies are exposed to the sun, we produce vitamin D, important for protecting our bones and warding off osteoporosis. Sun rays also benefit our sleep cycles and mood.

21 PAMPER YOURSELF
Manicures are a great way to feel glamorous. Choose a bright red color if you're feeling bold or a soft pink for a more understated look. Treat yourself to a full-body massage and take mental notes, then put them to good use later and offer your partner their own rubdown.

22 GET A HAIRCUT
Need a change, but not sure where to start? A haircut is the perfect way to switch up your style and feel amazing. In fact, you should try to get a haircut every 5-7 weeks to ensure healthy locks and avoid breakage.

23 WATCH A HAPPY MOVIE
Watching a film that gives you a warm, fuzzy feeling inside is an easy way to improve your mood.

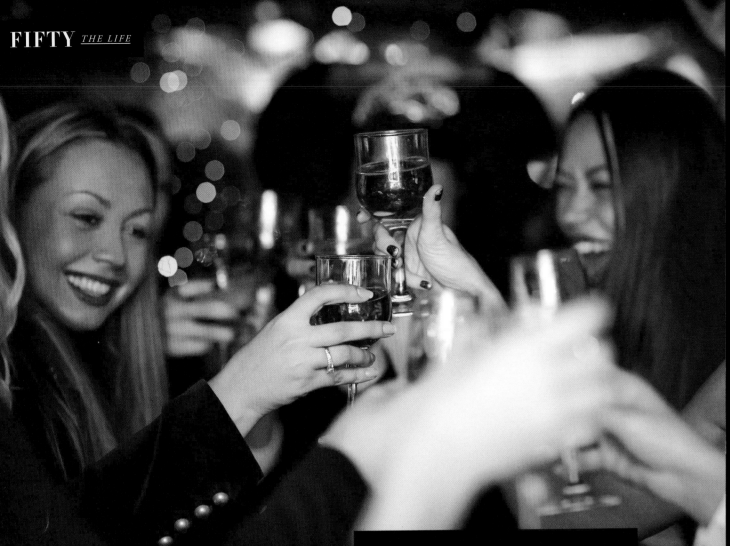

BE A SOCIAL BUTTERFLY

Human beings are social creatures, so don't be timid. Put yourself out there and embrace your confident inner goddess.

24 HIT HAPPY HOUR WITH WORK FRIENDS
Socializing can not only boost camaraderie, but it can further your career. Experts claim occasionally attending happy hour is an excellent way to show the boss you're a team player, and it will help you manage your reputation at work. Bottoms up!

25 VISIT WITH A FRIEND
There are hidden benefits to having supportive friends. One study found people with social support have fewer cardiovascular problems, immunity issues and lower levels of cortisol, a stress hormone. So unplug for a bit and visit in person rather than via text.

26 CALL YOUR PARENTS
According to attachment theorists, the relationship you share with your parents can play a huge role in other adult relationships. Plus, they brought you into the world,

ANA TALKED TO HER SUBCONSCIOUS 77 TIMES. WHEN IN DOUBT, WHY NOT REACH OUT TO A FRIEND?

so take the time to call at least once a week to keep them up to date on your life and to check in on theirs. If you live close by, pop by for a visit and catch up.

27 GO ON A BLIND DATE
Remember that "perfect match" your friend has been begging you to meet? Now's the time to take them up on the offer. Studies show women with a healthy dating life have higher self-esteem. Plus, there's the added benefit of falling in love (or at least setting standards for future relationships). So dig out your little black dress, and get out there and paint the town.

28 HAVE A GIRLS' NIGHT OUT
Friends aren't just good for the soul, they're good for your health. One study found being around close female friends can increase feelings of contentment. When you're with friends, the mood-elevating hormone oxytocin is released, which increases feelings of euphoria.

GET NATURALLY BEAUTIFUL

Feel better by treating your body to wholesome products you can make.

29 MAKE A MASK
Want clean, rejuvenated skin without having to go to the store? Look no further than your pantry or refrigerator for all you need to make a great face mask. Mix a teaspoon of oatmeal, a teaspoon of plain, live active yogurt and a few drops of warm honey. Apply to your face and rinse off with warm water after 10 minutes.

30 SHINE UP YOUR MANE
For truly radiant locks, combine mashed avocado with some coconut milk. Comb it through the hair and let it sit for 10 to 15 minutes before rinsing. The final step? Flaunt your gorgeous 'do!

31 MAKE AN ORANGE SCRUB
Have dry skin? Here's a quick fix that's all-natural and easy: Mix the juice of half an orange and four tablespoons of cornmeal into a paste. Apply to your freshly washed face and body, scrub and glow. You'll feel like a brand new person!

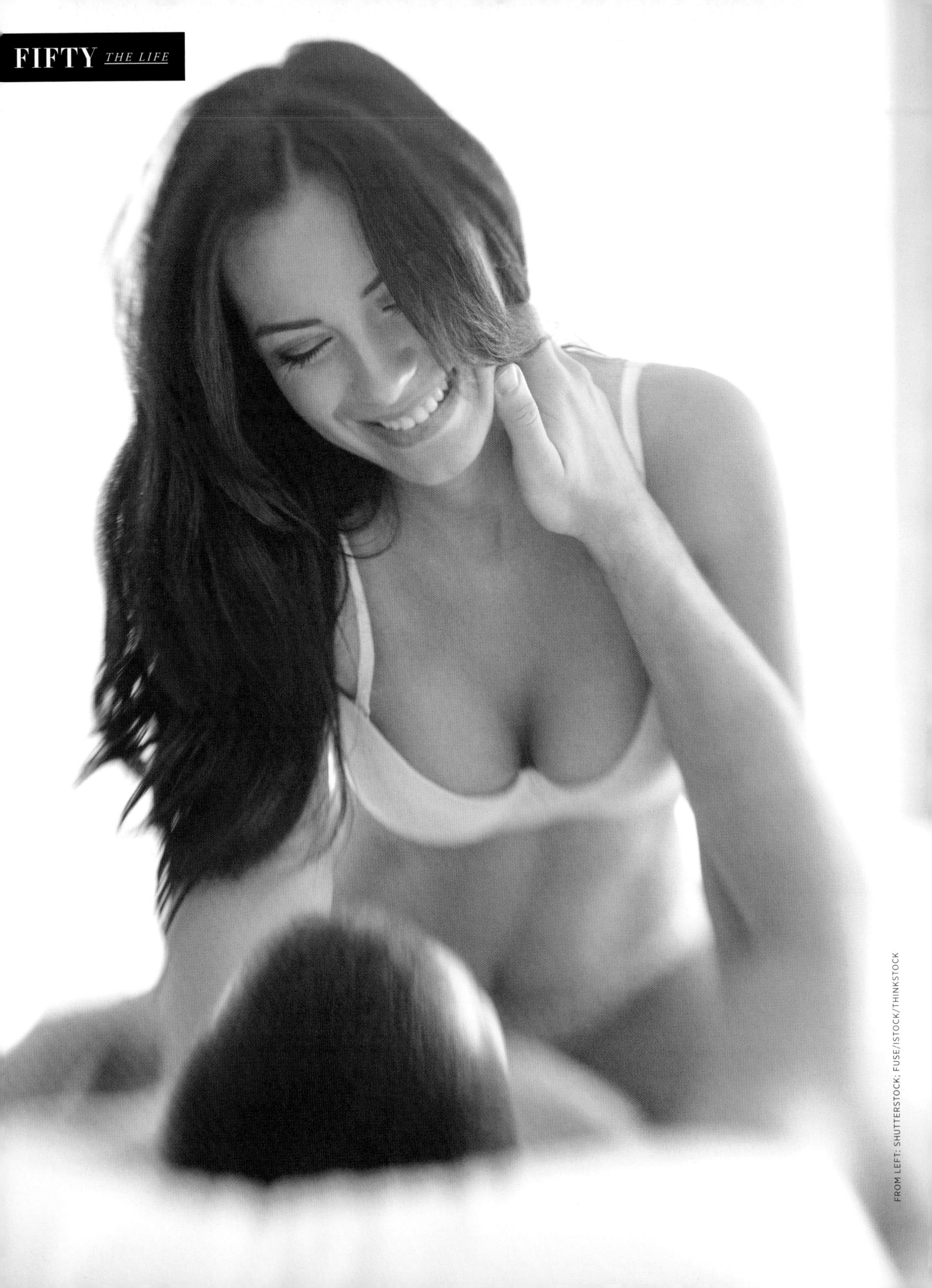

FROM LEFT: SHUTTERSTOCK; FUSE/ISTOCK/THINKSTOCK

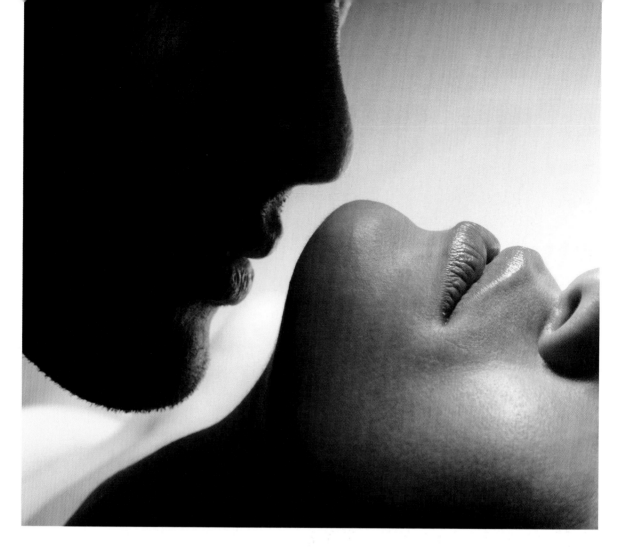

SEXPLORE YOURSELF

"I usually encourage women to independently explore what brings them pleasure and then bring that knowledge to their partner." —Dr. Villarreal

32 GET COMFORTABLE WITH YOURSELF
For a satisfying sex life, according to Dr. Villarreal, it's important to be comfortable in your own skin. So strip down and look in the mirror. You're unique and beautiful, so tell yourself that. Repeat it loudly and with confidence.

33 ENJOY YOUR BODY
Self-pleasuring is an important way to get in touch with your body, and research shows it can even improve your mood. Plus it helps to know what you like so you can teach your partner how to blow your mind.

34 OPEN A DIALOGUE
Toys in the bedroom are a great way to zest up your sex life. Dr. Jozkowski suggests revealing such desires to your partner in a non-threatening environment, such as over dinner. They'll quickly be hungry for more than their meal.

35 COMMEND YOURSELF FOR A JOB WELL DONE IN BED
Pat yourself on the back when you've pleased your partner. You've earned it! Recognizing sexual prowess is empowering and builds great confidence.

36 CREATE A PLAYLIST
Eager to try something new with your partner, but having trouble creating the right atmosphere? Create a playlist of 20 songs that get you in the mood and then see how far you get through the songs.

37 GET PLAYFUL
Sexual enhancement products like vibrators and body balms can be a fun way to spice up bedroom behavior. Or grab a tie and act out your favorite scenes from *Fifty Shades*.

38 SPRUCE UP YOUR STYLE WITH NEW LINGERIE
Lingerie is a covert way to feel sexy. Buy yourself a bra and panty set you feel amazing in, and slip them under your daily wardrobe. You'll sport an instant glow, knowing what's hiding underneath.

39 GET HONEST
"Sex isn't talked about as often as it could be for women to feel fulfilled sexually," says Dr. Villarreal. So sit down with your partner and share all your favorite things in bed to achieve peak pleasure! Encourage them to open up about their likes and dislikes as well.

40 BE OPEN TO NEW THINGS
According to Dr. Jozkowski, willingness to try new things with your partner can aid a relationship on the rocks. So take out a copy of *Fifty Shades of Grey*, read it aloud with your mate and discuss the parts that turn you on.

DO GOOD DEEDS

Take a note from Christian and help others. You'll feel good about yourself, and feeling better about you is the essence of self-satisfaction.

41 VOLUNTEER
Reports have shown that those who volunteer have greater longevity, lower rates of depression and fewer incidences of heart disease. Check out *homelessshelterdirectory.org* to find out where you can lend a hand at a local homeless shelter.

42 DONATE CLOTHING
Remember the pile of clothes in the back of your closet that you never wear? Check out *use.salvationarmy.org* to find out where you can donate your extra clothing.

43 WORK WITH ANIMALS
It's estimated that 7.6 million companion animals enter shelters every year. Visit *petfinder.com/shelters* to find a shelter and make a difference.

44 WALK FOR A CAUSE
Thanks to the combined efforts of about 150,000 Avon Walk participants since 2003, more than $500 million has been raised and donated to breast cancer programs.

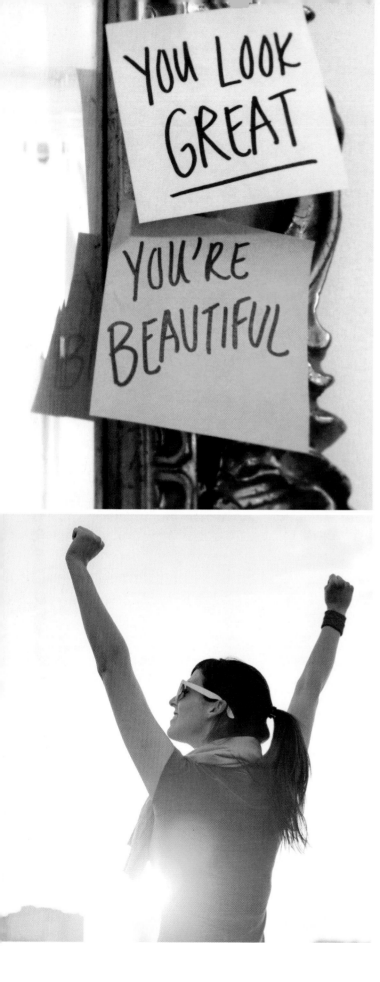

CHANGE YOUR ATTITUDE

A positive outlook often leads to a positive outcome, in the boardroom and in the bedroom.

45 GIVE A COMPLIMENT
"A lot of women don't feel confident and feel insecure about their weight, their looks, their body size or even their genitals," says Dr. Jozkowski. Want to get an instant beauty boost, without an ounce of makeup? Give your best friend a call and let her know how beautiful she is. You'll make her day, and you'll feel amazing too.

46 SHIFT PERSPECTIVE
Instead of asking yourself, "How good can I look?" Dr. Jozkowski suggests asking yourself, "How good can I feel?" After all, beauty radiates from the inside out.

47 RECOGNIZE THAT YOU DESERVE PLEASURE
Psychologists claim that acknowledging you are deserving of pleasure is a key element to feeling fulfilled and happy. So give yourself the OK, and enjoy yourself shamelessly.

48 MAKE A LIST OF POSITIVE QUALITIES
Make a list of all your favorite things about yourself including skills, experiences, body parts, personality traits and anything else about you that makes you feel good. Add to the list the compliments others have given you as well. Reminding yourself of your assets is a confidence booster, and confidence is sexy.

49 GET SPIRITUAL
Studies indicate meditation can lead to lower levels of stress and anxiety, which can ultimately diminish the probability of heart disease. Also, teaching your mind to switch off from the worries that build up during the day is immensely therapeutic. Beginners can start with five minutes of meditation and increase as they feel more comfortable.

50 THANK YOUR BODY
According to Dr. Jozkowski, it is essential to thank your body after you've done something positive for it. Whether you've completed a two-hour hot yoga class, a three-mile run, a spinning class or a wholesome bowl of oatmeal and berries, thank yourself for being kind to your body. This positive reinforcement is key to releasing your inner goddess.

....

**Kristen Jozkowski, assistant professor of Community Health Promotion at the University of Arkansas
Dr. Christina Villarreal maintains a private psychotherapy and forensic assessment practice in Oakland, California**

BUNS OF STEELE

One simple and effective exercise to whip you into sex-goddess shape.

If you're anything like Ana, then working out is not on your daily to-do list. But just as she negotiates her way out of exercising more than she has to, women everywhere spend more time talking themselves out of hitting the gym than it takes to actually get there. This kettlebell routine can be done quickly and easily at home. Plus, it's the perfect challenge for your body to build strength, increase stamina and promote flexibility.

EXERCISE 1
Targets: Quads, glutes, abs

1. Spread your legs shoulder-width apart, holding the kettlebell at chest height.
2. Bend your knees and sit back as if you were preparing to sit in a chair. Keep your eyes focused forward and tighten your core to ensure your back remains straight. Your thighs should be parallel to the ground.
3. Stand up and repeat the exercise 10 to 20 times.

3

10 LBS

Bell Curves
Make sure to choose a kettlebell that's the proper weight for your body. Many trainers suggest women begin with an 18-pound kettlebell, but beginner kettlebells are available at weights as low as six pounds.

EXERCISE 2

Targets: Arms, shoulders, back

1. Stand with your feet a bit wider than shoulder width with a slight bend in your knee. Grab the kettlebell handle with one hand.
2. Swing the kettlebell out and away from your body until your arm is fully extended. Make sure to control the kettlebell so it won't swing over your head. It should end up near your shoulder height.
3. As gravity pulls it back down, return to your start position and allow the kettlebell to swing backward between your legs. Do 15 reps with each arm.

EXERCISE 3

Targets: Quads, glutes, shoulders

1. As with the first exercise, stand with your legs shoulder-width apart. Hold the kettlebell in front with both hands.
2. Step forward with your right leg into a lunge until your thigh is parallel with the ground, pulling the kettlebell up to your chest with elbows pointed out. Hold and pulse for 10 counts. Make sure your knee does not touch the floor.
3. Step back, returning to your original position and repeat with your left leg. Do each leg 10 times.

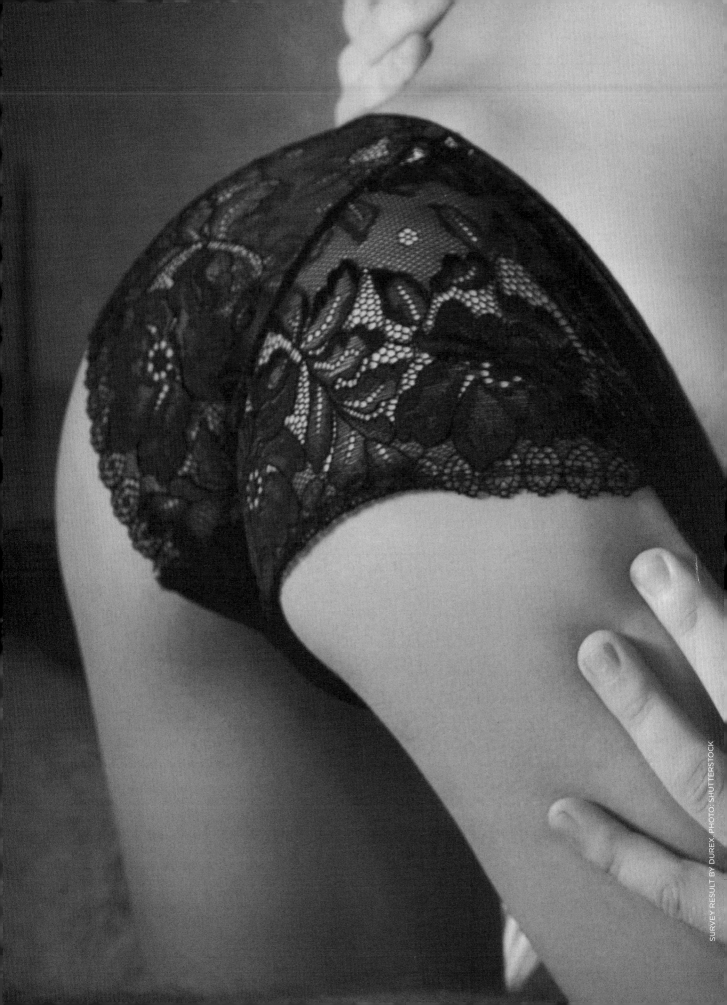

*75% **of women** never reach their "peak"* **through sex alone.**

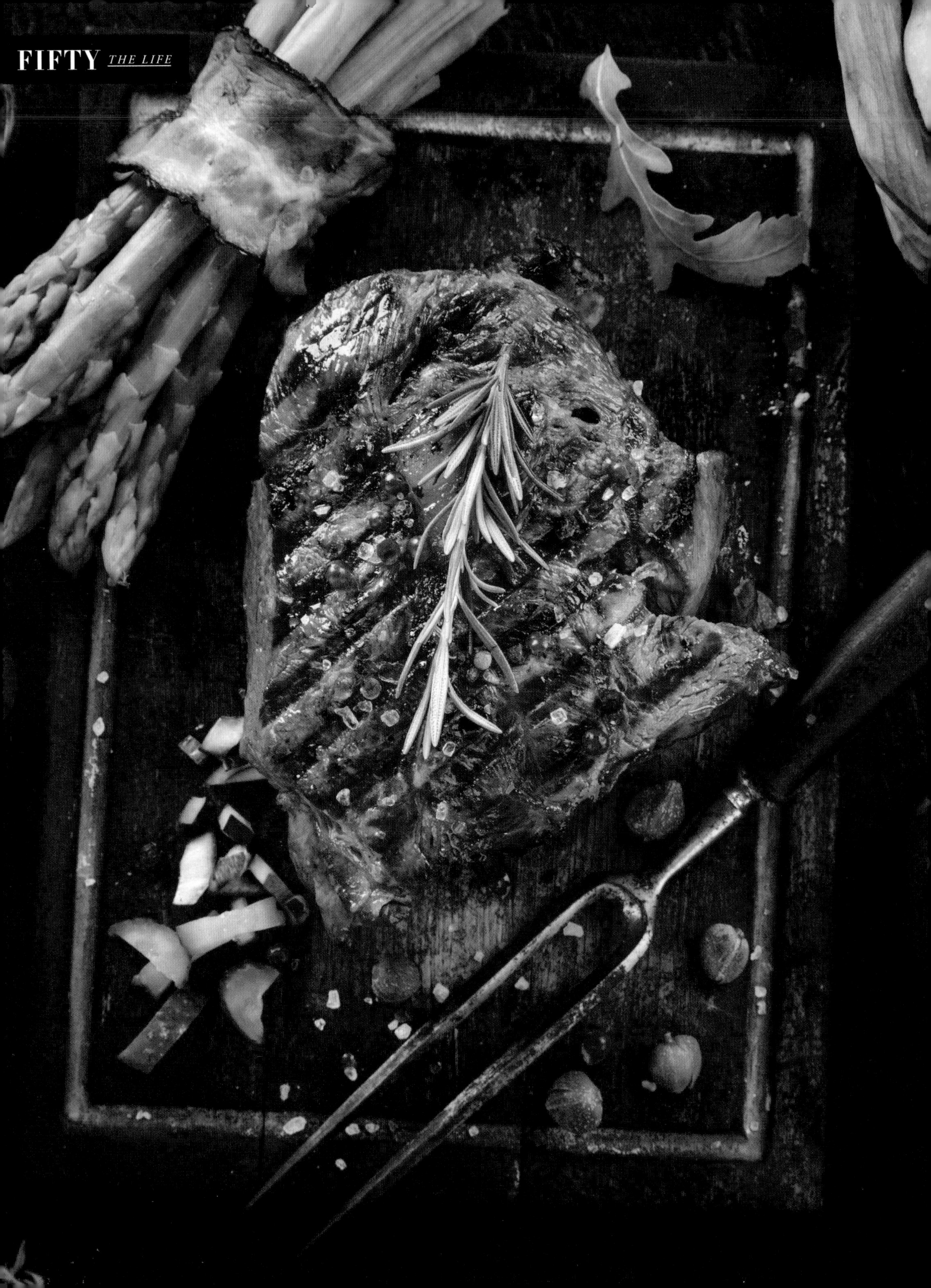

FIFTY SHADES OF FOOD

Some of the most erotic passages from the *Fifty Shades* trilogy don't describe sex—they detail the meals enjoyed by the story's main characters. Here's how to make some of them yourself.

◀ LEMON AND GARLIC MARINATED STEAK

The simple steak served at Bob's in the first book gets tweaked with some cilantro and soy sauce.

- **1** flank steak (1.2–1.5 lbs)
- **1** tablespoon olive oil
- **2** teaspoons soy sauce
- **2** teaspoons lemon juice (fresh squeezed)
- **3** garlic cloves, chopped
- **¼** cup chopped cilantro
  Fresh ground sea salt and pepper to taste

1. Combine ingredients in glass dish and let marinate for several hours.

2. Light gas grill on medium-high heat. Cook steaks for about 8–10 minutes for medium rare (4–5 minutes per side depending on thickness).

3. Let steak rest for 10 minutes.

4. Slice meat against the grain in thin slices and serve.

STRAWBERRY DAIQUIRIS

This refreshing summer drink is perfect for loosening inhibitions and unleashing your inner goddess. It certainly did the trick for Ana.

- **1** cup white rum
- **⅓** cup Grand Marnier
- **3** cups fresh strawberries, hulled and roughly chopped
- **¼** cup fresh-squeezed lime juice
- **1–1½** cups sugar
  Ice cubes

1. In a blender, combine the rum, Grand Marnier, strawberries, fresh-squeezed lime juice and one cup of ice.

2. Add additional ½ cup of ice to reach desired consistency.

3. Pour gently into sugar-rimmed glasses.

OYSTERS

One of Ana's many firsts with Christian, the raw oyster's abundance of sex-hormone producing amino acids make it a classic aphrodisiac. Purists maintain you need to eat them raw, but there's nothing wrong with a little mignonette sauce to add some pep.

- 1 tablespoon coarsely ground white or black peppercorns for a little heat—to taste
- ½ cup white or red wine vinegar
- 2 tablespoons finely chopped shallots

  Salt to taste

1. Combine all ingredients and chill. Serve with chilled oysters or clams on the half shell.

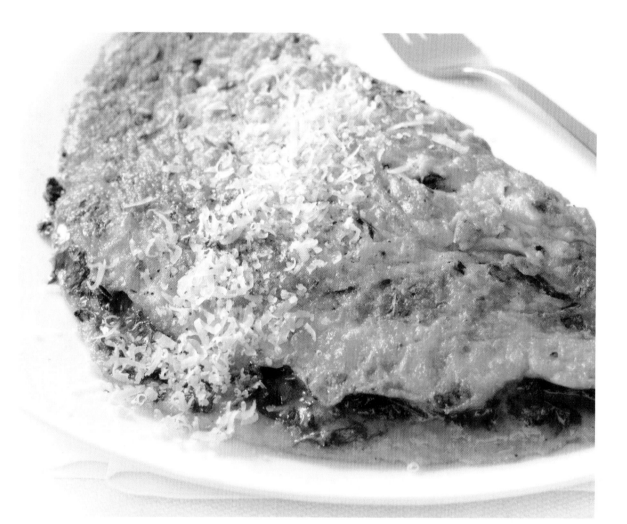

MUSHROOM, SPINACH AND CHEESE OMELETTE

Starting your day with this healthy breakfast served to Ana by Mrs. Jones in *Fifty Shades Freed* means you can later indulge in plenty of bad habits, food-related or otherwise.

Olive oil to coat
the pan

1 tablespoon chopped
shallots

8 button mushrooms,
thinly sliced

2 cups baby spinach

½ tablespoon butter

2 eggs

2 egg whites

3 tablespoons
low-fat milk

3 tablespoons
fresh mozzarella,
thinly sliced

Salt, pepper and
garlic powder to taste

1. Heat a nonstick 8-inch or well-seasoned heavy steel skillet over medium-high heat for 1 minute. Add enough olive oil to lightly coat the pan.

2. Add mushrooms and sauté until browned (about 5–6 minutes).

3. Add shallots and sauté for 2 minutes longer until softened.

4. Stir in spinach and sauté for 1 minute until spinach begins to wilt.

5. Season spinach and mushroom mixture with salt, pepper and a bit of garlic powder. Remove from pan and set aside.

6. Add ½ tablespoon butter to pan until butter begins to sizzle.

7. Beat eggs, egg whites and milk and pour into pan. Cook the egg mixture for approximately 1–2 minutes, pulling up the edges with a heatproof silicone spatula to allow the uncooked eggs to run into the center of the pan. Cook for up to 1 minute longer until the eggs begin to set.

8. Add fresh mozzarella and spinach mixture to one half of the egg.

9. Using the spatula, fold up ⅓ of the omelette. Roll the omelette over onto itself, then tilt the pan and slide omelette onto a plate. Let sit for an extra minute until cheese is melted and serve.

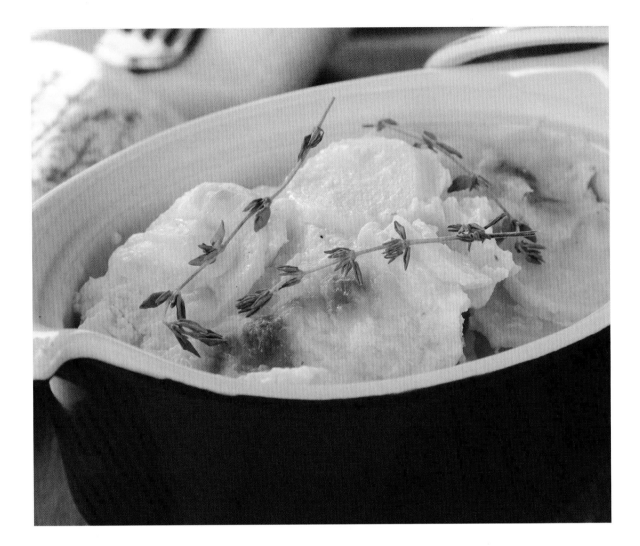

DAUPHINOISE POTATOES

It'll take a few sessions in the Red Room of Pain to burn off these rich and luxurious potatoes served in *Fifty Shades Freed*. The fennel and shallot add a twist to the classic dish.

2 small fennel bulbs

1 shallot, thinly sliced

2 tablespoons olive oil

1 tablespoon salted butter

2 pounds Yukon Gold potatoes, thinly sliced

2 cups plus 2 tablespoons heavy cream

2½ cups grated Gruyère (approximately ½ lb)

1 teaspoon sea salt

½ teaspoon freshly ground black pepper

1. Preheat oven to 350°.

2. Butter a 10 x 15 x 2 baking dish.

3. Remove stalks of fennel and cut in half lengthwise. Remove bulbs and slice very thinly, making approximately 4 cups of sliced fennel. Thinly slice the shallot.

4. Sauté the fennel and shallot with olive oil and butter on medium-low heat for 15 minutes until very tender.

5. Peel the potatoes, then thinly slice them with a mandoline or by hand (should be less than ⅛ of an inch thick). Mix the sliced potatoes in a large bowl with 2 cups of cream, 2 cups of Gruyère, salt and pepper. Add the fennel and shallot and mix well.

6. Pour the potatoes into the dish and press on the potatoes to smooth out. Mix the remaining 2 tablespoons of cream and ½ cup of Gruyère and sprinkle on the top.

7. Bake for 1½ hours. Potatoes will be very tender, bubbly and browned. Let sit for 10-15 minutes to cool and serve.

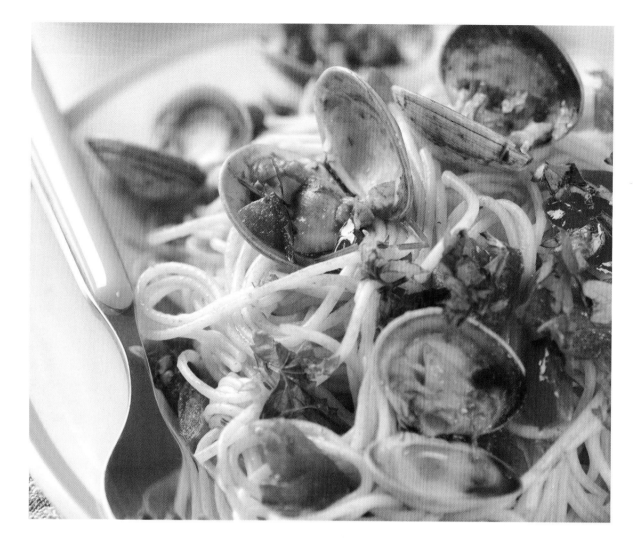

PASTA ALLE VONGOLE

This pasta dish served with a white wine sauce and fresh clams makes a perfect light dinner if you're planning to engage in some strenuous physical activity later on. It's a dish that Mrs. Jones serves to Christian often, and one that'll soon become one of your favorites too.

2 lbs fresh clams (Manila or Littleneck)

1 package spaghetti

2 tablespoons butter

2 tablespoons olive oil

3-4 garlic cloves, chopped

1 teaspoon red pepper flakes

½ cup dry white wine

2 tablespoons fresh parsley, chopped

1 teaspoon lemon zest

10 cherry tomatoes, halved

Salt and pepper to taste

1. Rinse clams in cold water, scrubbing as necessary. Put in a large bowl and cover with cold water. Salt and let sit in water for at least an hour (preferably a few). Drain and rinse, removing any sand or grit.

2. Cook spaghetti in a large pot of salted boiling water as recommended by directions until al dente.

3. Put half the butter and olive oil in a large pan over medium heat until sizzling. Add red pepper flakes and garlic. Cook until garlic softens.

4. Add the white wine to the garlic and bring to a boil. Add clams and a few squeezes of lemon and cover the pan. Stir periodically to ensure the clams get a sufficient amount of heat. Clams should open in approximately 4 minutes. Discard any that have not opened.

5. Drain spaghetti and add to the pan along with remaining butter. Toss well and let sit for one minute.

6. Add parsley, lemon zest, cherry tomatoes and a squirt of lemon, season with salt and pepper to taste and serve.

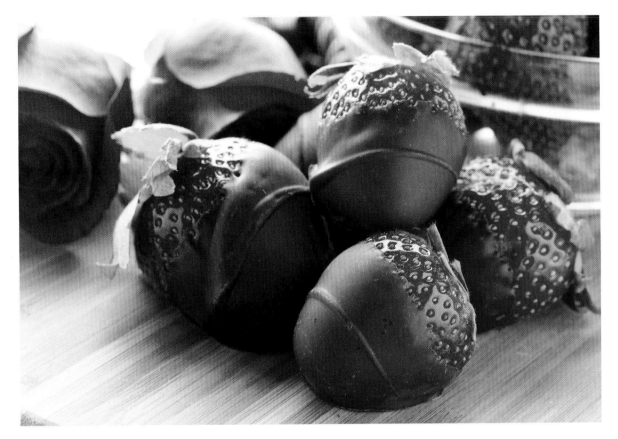

▲ CHOCOLATE-COVERED STRAWBERRIES

Chocolate is considered the king of all aphrodisiacs because of its dual ability to physically relax the body while simultaneously increasing dopamine levels directly related to orgasm intensity.

- 2 tablespoons sugar
- 1 cup heavy cream
- 8 ounces chopped bittersweet chocolate
- 1 tablespoon butter
- 1 tablespoon Cabernet Sauvignon
  Pound cake cubes
  Strawberries, cleaned
  Bits of ginger cookie or biscotti

1. In a microwave-safe bowl, mix the sugar, heavy cream, chocolate and butter together. Microwave for 2 minutes.

2. Take out of microwave, add wine and whisk.

3. Transfer to either a fondue pot with a flame underneath or a double boiler.

4. Serve with pound cake cubes, strawberries and biscotti bits for dipping.

LEMON SYLLABUB ▶

Don't let the lemons fool you. This dessert, enjoyed at a Grey family dinner, will be the sweetest thing you eat all week. Month. Year.

- ⅓ cup lemon juice (strained)
- ¼ cup Scotch whisky
- 1 tablespoon lemon zest
- ¼ cup superfine sugar
- 1 cup heavy cream
- ¼ teaspoon nutmeg
  Berries for topping (optional)

1. Mix lemon juice, Scotch whisky and lemon zest and let sit for 4–6 hours.

2. Whip the cream with the sugar in a separate bowl until cream begins to form peaks. Gradually add the lemon/whisky mixture. Whip until light and fluffy, not grainy.

3. Serve in chilled glasses and sprinkle nutmeg on top along with fresh berries (optional).

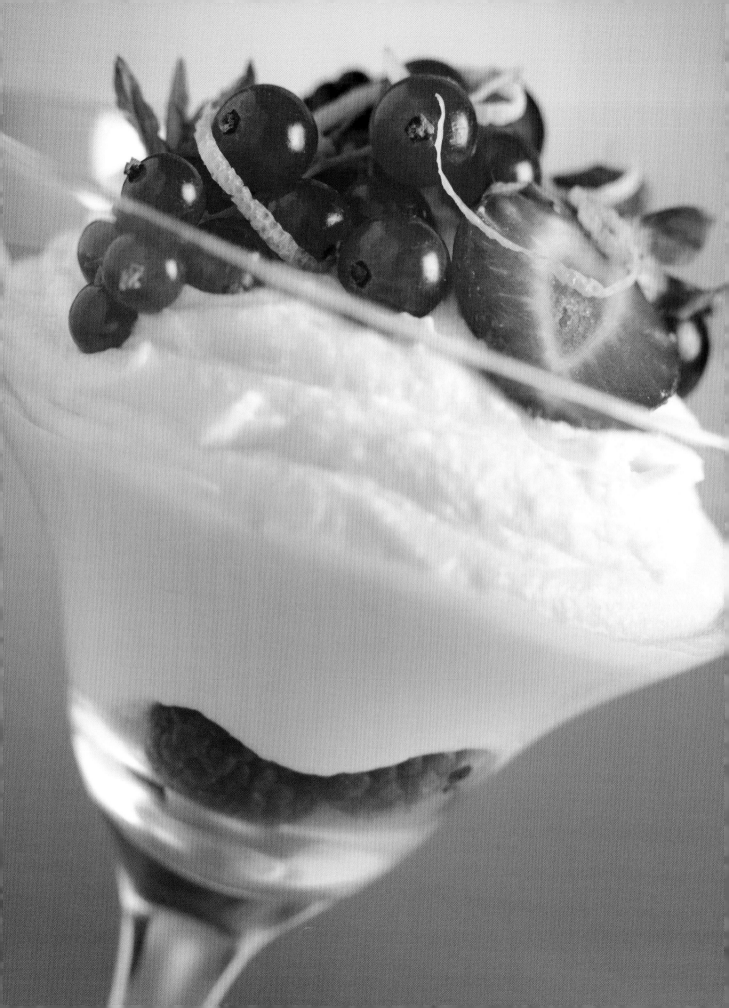

Though Seattle is the famous backdrop for Fifty, women fantasize about being intimate at the Eiffel Tower, while men fantasize about the White House.

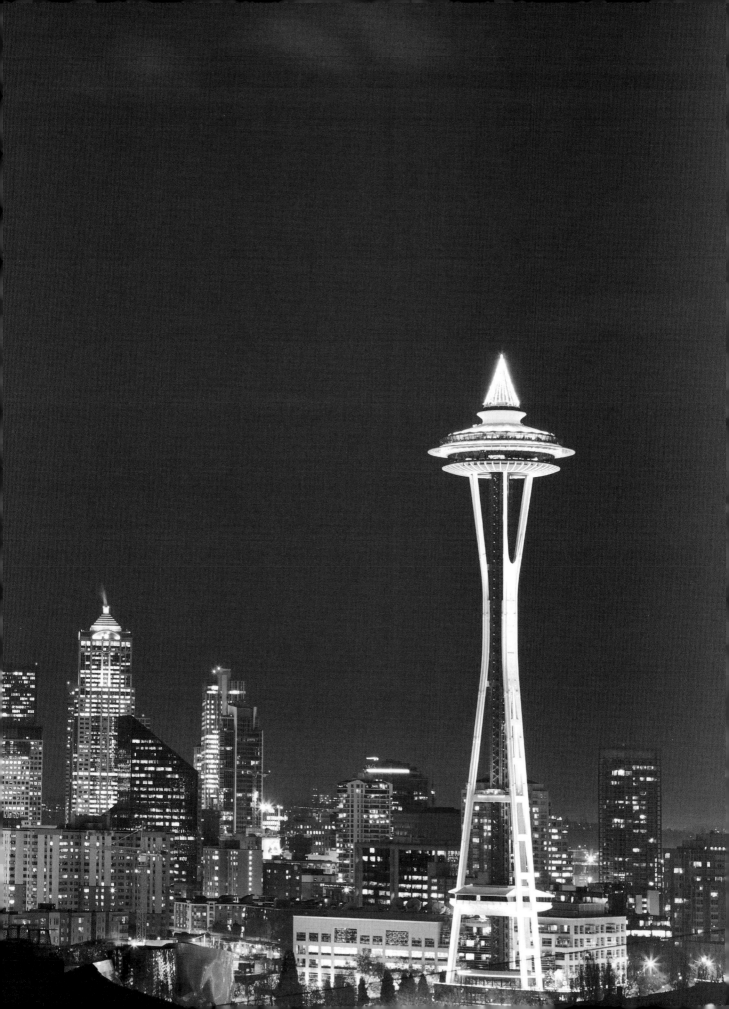

HOW TO HAVE HOTTER SEX

Dr. Carol Queen of Good Vibrations, a San Francisco-based sex toy store, shares secrets that will take you from blushing novice to full-blown sexpert.

DO THE RESEARCH

"Whether it's with toys or something else in the bedroom, it never hurts to read about it. You can learn about toys just by going online and finding the blogs of toy reviews. Goodvibes.com has reviews from users and buyers, so people can see what others think."

BE POSITIVE

"It's possible to have a sex talk that doesn't open with 'I'm unsatisfied with our sex life.' Be reassuring. 'I love what we do, I love the way we have sex, I especially love this, this and this,' but follow that up with 'Gosh, I'm so curious about this, is there anything you're curious about?'"

GET BACK ON THE BIKE

"Realize that the first kinky thing you try might not be your favorite thing, just like your first time with sex might not have been the best ever. But you keep trying. If you had a less than stellar experience with something, it doesn't hurt to try it again."

Whether you've been with your loved one for 50 days or 50 years, it's likely, and often recommended, that you spice things up in the bedroom every once in awhile to reignite that spark between you—or at least keep it burning. Millions have turned to *Fifty Shades of Grey* for help, and for good reason. It's catapulted its way from simple, sexy novel to sexual playbook for couples everywhere, inciting and inspiring people to try something new. So if it's whips and floggers, roleplaying or just an open conversation, Dr. Queen offers quick tips for improving your sex life.

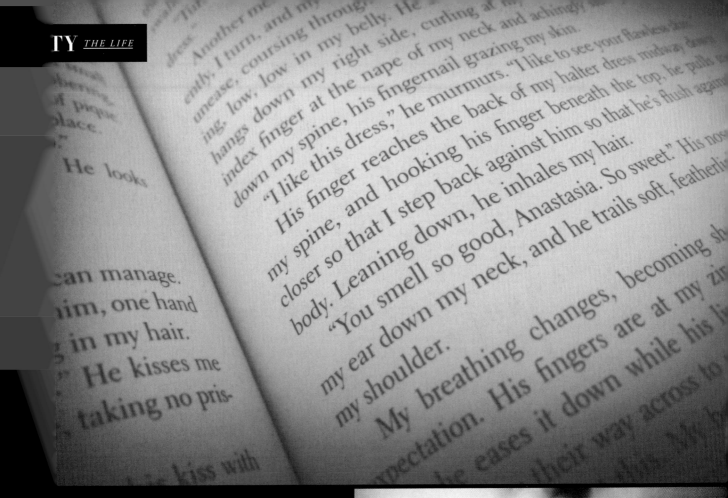

Another me... gently, I turn, and my... ease, coursing through... ing, low, low in my belly. He... hangs down my right side, curling at... index finger at the nape of my neck and aching... down my spine, his fingernail grazing my skin.

"I like this dress," he murmurs. "I like to see your flawless...

His finger reaches the back of my halter dress midway down... my spine, and hooking his finger beneath the top, he pulls me... closer so that I step back against him so that he's flush again... body. Leaning down, he inhales my hair.

"You smell so good, Anastasia. So sweet." His no... my ear down my neck, and he trails soft, featherli... my shoulder.

My breathing changes, becoming sh... ...pectation. His fingers are at my zi... ...e eases it down while his li... ...their way across to...

He looks... can manage... ...im, one hand... ...g in my hair.

He kisses me... taking no pris-... ...e kiss with...

BE BOLD

'It might not feel normal for you to say, 'Hey honey, I had a sexual fantasy...' But showing your partner a passage from *Fifty Shades* for example and saying, 'Do you think this is intriguing too?' 's not so different from saying, 'Wow, did you see his wild thing this politician said today?'"

IMPROVISE

"Role-play is an attractive and powerful way to have erotic experiences. You don't have to say, 'Oh can't do that, I'm too shy...' You can pretend to be someone like Anastasia, the curious virgin, and consider how she would respond."

BUY A TOY

'It's empowering for a woman to shop for a pleasure-related item. It's a way of saying 'sexual pleasure is important to me, and I'm going to see what's out there.' It turns out to be one of the most important experiences in terms of bringing out sexuality and confidence." Visit Good Vibrations, op right, or *goodvibes.com* for female-friendly and

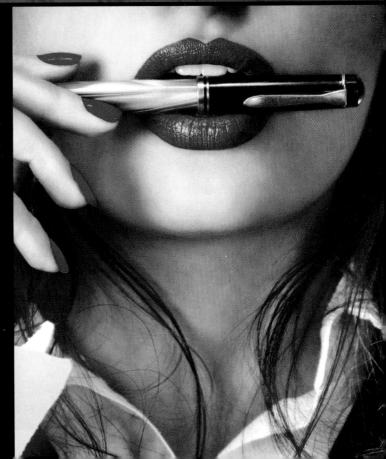

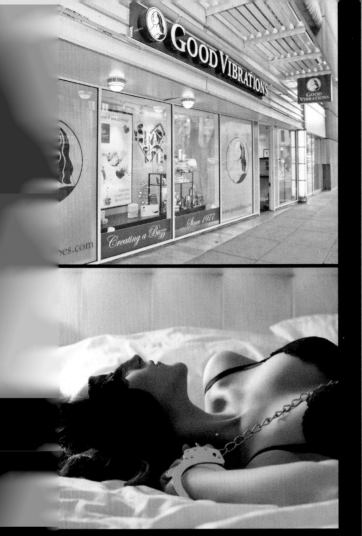

Positive Sex Energy
Left: Highlighting favorite passages from *Fifty Shades* and trying them out or bringing role-play into the bedroom are simple and fun ways to explore your sexuality with your partner. Top: Good Vibrations is a woman-focused sex toy retailer that strives to provide high-quality products and non-judgemental sex advice and education.

GIVE AND TAKE

'It's not inappropriate for couples to trade favorite experiences. If you like a little bondage, but he doesn't, compromise. 'We'll go to your favorite restaurant tonight, but tomorrow we're going to mine.' It's not like a couple has never negotiated before. They maybe just never have about sex. If neither of you want to be the dominant, make a deal: 'I'll spank you, but only if you spank me tomorrow.'"

TURN THE TABLES

"Try toys on him. Many guys have no idea they

SAFE TIPS FOR BEGINNERS

Follow this pro advice the next time you want to hit it off with your partner.

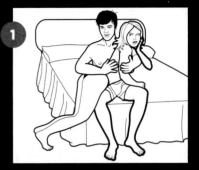

ASSUME THE POSITION
The spankee should be in a comfortable position over the lap of the spanker or on the bed.

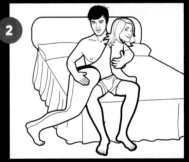

FEEL THINGS OUT
Don't just start whaling away. Some slow, sensual touching can calm a nervous partner and will definitely help set the mood.

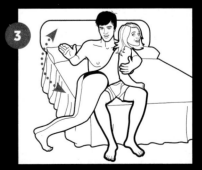

KEEP A LIGHT TOUCH
Light taps will prevent your partner from fleeing in terror and will build a sense of anticipation.

Women wait 6 months to 1 year before talking about sexual fantasies. Men wait just 3 months.